Fitz Koe

MY NOISY CANCE

Running at the Mouth, While Running for My Life

Fitzness Books
A division of Fitzness International LLC

Fitzness in a registered trademark of Fitz Koehler and Fitzness International LLC
Gainesville, FL

Koehler, Fitz
My Noisy Cancer Comeback: Running at the Mouth while Running for my Life

Fitzness International LLC non-fiction original hardcover
1. Biography & Autobiography – Women. 2. Health & Fitness – Diseases - Cancer
3. Sports & Recreation - Running & Jogging

Front cover photo by Rebecca Herrera
Back cover photos by Dianne Chan and Greg Sadler
Cover Designer: Alexander Von Ness
Layout Designer: Alen Čar - Slim Rijeka
Editor: Valeria Delgado

Contributing editors: Kristen Seymour, Rudy Novotny, Jennifer Senn, Eva Solomon,
Emily Thach, Lauren Gelman, and Eric Wendell

Proofreaders: Carla Engle and Doug Thurston

ISBN
978-1-7355998-1-6

MY NOISY CANCER COMEBACK

Running at the Mouth, while Running for my Life

By Fitz Koehler, M.S.E.S.S.

Fitzness Books

A division of Fitzness International LLC

Foreword

You never know when, where, or how we will meet them, the people that come into our lives and make a lasting impact. For me, that was in Orlando while I was announcing the 2013 runDisney races. There she was, this beautiful, blonde, blue-eyed girl with a smile as big as Texas. She dragged a booted leg over and introduced herself as Fitz Koehler. It is both fair and accurate to say that nothing has been the same since. I had no clue that Fitz would go on to become my favorite race announcer, partner, and best friend.

Fitz is an absolute dynamo of sincerity and energy. Her positive attitude is incredibly infectious and she is truly one of those people who has no bad days. And that's only because she doesn't allow them. At 5' 5", the girl is large and very much in charge. That's something I would come to know in short time.

Watching Fitz do public events and corporate presentations gave me an opportunity to see how comfortable she was with people. And, perhaps more importantly, how warmly they related to her. Having several decades of experience in an industry where working well with people is everything, I didn't think twice about recommending her for an opportunity to announce a major marathon weekend with me the following year. As it turns out, handing Fitz Koehler a microphone in front of nearly 20,000 adrenaline-fueled runners was one of the very best ideas

I've ever had. A star was born and we both realized this was her calling. Since then, Fitz has become among the most sought-after and respected event announcers in the country.

She is also one of the most gifted people I have ever known: intelligent, sarcastic, patriotic, fun, and funny. However, her most endearing quality is her genuine love for people—especially the sweaty ones. There are a number of fine race announcers, but few who take the time and effort to connect with their runners. Fitz consistently makes herself available on a personal and professional level, something that has created a very noisy and loyal following. Hordes of people think nothing of flying across the country to run her races.

As our friendship grew, I learned a lot about this badass kickboxer, fitness professional, and devoted mother. It was clear from the beginning that Fitz was someone determined to change the world for the better. Despite having a ton of projects and milestones under her belt, she would be the first to tell you that she's "just getting started!" To say that she has a passion for getting and keeping people fit would be an insane understatement. Millions have learned to make better food choices and fitness decisions through her guidance.

Fitz's 2019 schedule was packed with events, many of which we would be announcing together, and she made it abundantly clear that she wouldn't even consider taking time off. The first time I witnessed her resolve was at our largest event of the year, The Los Angeles Marathon. It was a mere 11 days after receiving her first round of chemotherapy. As we welcomed 25,000 athletes through the finish line, the evidence that the brutal drugs were taking a toll on my friend was everywhere. Long, beautiful, blonde hair covered our black stage floor. Still, Fitz gave no less than 100-percent. Her joyful voice could be heard all morning welcoming athletes "home."

As she charged forward with grace and determination, I would go on to learn more about Fitz. I watched her struggle to walk short distances and endure medical treatments just to stay upright for announcing. It was shocking to see her knocked down repeatedly. But she always hoisted herself back up and never once complained.

To be thrust into the public eye while not looking or feeling your best would make even the bravest retreat. But my noisy BFF charged forward with television interviews, fitness presentations, and races almost every weekend.

When Fitz told me that she was writing a book, I knew it would be captivating--and not just because I watched her live it. When I read her manuscript, I was touched that she shared so many raw moments. Cancer is terrifying, but rather than dwell on that, her novel reveals the darkest days with a light, never-ending smile. She found a way to address the shocking and strange side of her experiences in a comical way—giving new meaning to the words wig, sludge, and ogre (you'll know what I'm talking about soon). Her snarky take on the big C made me laugh. A lot. I beamed with pride while reading about her defiantly announcing races across the country, often days before or after undergoing chemotherapy. Was I surprised? No. That's just the badass my Team Noisy partner is (you'll learn about that too).

Her victory over this horrible disease is an entertaining and educational story. And whether you're a runner, one of her Hotties, a fellow Gator, a cancer warrior, or simply someone looking for some inspiration, I believe you will enjoy the journey ahead. And I know you will come away with an awesome degree of respect and a better understanding of what it takes to accept, endure, and overcome such a challenge.

Rudy Novotny
Race Announcer
Sub 3-Hour Marathoner
Celebrator of the Human Spirit

Contents

This book is dedicated to those who funded, conducted, and implemented the research that saved my life.

Chapter 1

Life at Full Volume

Standing on stages bald and sick was never on my to-do list, but doing so was a hell of a lot better than being stuck in the hospital or six feet under. And it also came with incredible power. In fact, I was stunned by my ability to hush crowds of 10,000+ with the simple act of removing my hat. "Oh, my God, she's bald! Oh no. I think she has cancer." It ran through the minds of everyone in my audience and I used that attention and concern to do what I've always done: compel others to take their own health seriously. I could have taken the year off and everyone would have understood. Everyone, that is, but me. Breast cancer tried to take me down, so I fought tooth and nail to stand the hell up. I fought for my life, I fought for my family, and I fought for the career that I adored.

Everyone loves a good comeback story. Well, at least most people do. And, in my not-so-humble opinion, noisy comeback stories are the best. As I write this, I feel like I must continuously knock on wood, because getting too cocky and noisy about beating cancer seems like I'm asking for trouble. However, without taunting the big bully who invaded my left boob, I think it's fair to tell the tale. My tale.

I'm writing this on the other side of breast cancer, but still living in the Twilight Zone. As a close spectator while family and friends have gone through it, I've always respected the misery that cancer and its treatment could inflict. However, I never fully comprehended all of the minutiae: the weird, painful, stressful, or even comical side effects and scenarios that a patient must endure while trying to survive. In fact, those weird things are kind of what inspired me to write this book.

When the side effects of my treatment started kicking in, each day brought a new "What the Hell" moment. The kind of stuff you just can't make up. And, on top of dealing with a nuclear bomb's worth of side effects from chemotherapy, radiation, and surgery, I was traveling all over the United States almost every weekend. I was deathly ill at

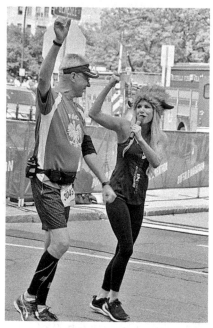

Buffalo Marathon finish line.
May 27, 2018.
Photo by: Darell McKenrick

points, but I never let that interfere with announcing some of the largest and most prestigious running events in the country. In order to hide my struggles from the runners, race directors, spectators, and friends in attendance, I went to some pretty extreme measures. I also implemented some fairly odd tactics just to remain upright.

My experience wasn't quick or easy as some people suggested it might be — it was brutal. Every cell in my body was being ravaged. And I felt it. But the last thing I wanted to be, or allow people to view me as, was a victim. Strength, power, and grittiness are my favorite qualities to find in others, and they're certainly the things I love most about myself. So I decided instead, to be a victor. In the face of a potentially lethal disease, I chose to maintain a positive outlook. I chose to smile and laugh when I could. I chose not to whine … EVER. I chose a relentless pursuit of my career and quality time with my loved ones. And, when cancer treatment was tearing me limb from limb, I chose not to share that publicly. I wasn't simply trying to trick people, I just couldn't handle the emotional toll revealing my suffering would have yielded. I also had no interest in giving cancer any glory; I was going to get the better of it, not the other way around. Continuing to project strength and joy was something I could control, so I did. And it was very empowering.

It's still very difficult to wrap my head around the fact that I *actually* had cancer. I also can't believe that I had chemo, radiation, and surgeries. That stuff only happens to other people, right? Apparently not. Breast cancer happened to me. And if it happened to me, it can happen to anybody. I won my battle for two reasons: excellent medical care and purpose. I will thank scientists, medical practitioners, and those who fund them for the rest of my days. They literally saved my life. But purpose...that was all me. Before my diagnosis I had created a spectacular life with a career I was passionate about, people I cared about, and a huge list of things to live for. This was my driving force. I hope by the end of this book, you'll evaluate your reason for being and make sure it's one worth fighting for.

Now that cancer is in my rearview mirror, I'm ready to share my fairly juicy story — one that's filled with all the gory details about the an-

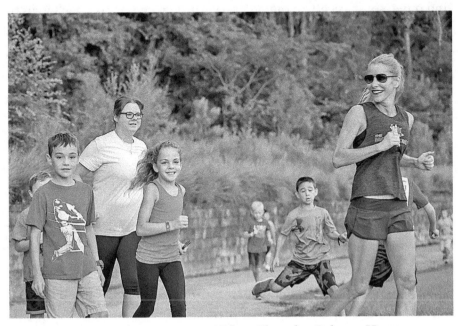

Running with my Morning Milers. Photo by: Rebecca Herrera

gry little cell that tried to silence this very noisy and very bossy blonde. Before I get to the nitty-gritty details about the Big C, I'll backtrack just a little bit so you know where I was in the life I had previously. It was both pretty basic and kind of extraordinary at the same time. At home in Gainesville, Florida, I spent my days as a wife, mother, animal lover, and business owner. Rob, my husband of 20 years, is a police lieutenant who's smart, funny, and so handsome that his nickname on the street is "pretty boy." He's the ultimate gentleman who knows no other way than to give 1,000% to every task he undertakes. Our daughter Ginger, 16 at the time of my diagnosis, is the spitting image of me, but better. I often call her Fitz 2.0 - the new and improved version! She's exactly my height, almost 5'6", has beautiful long blonde hair, and sparkly blue eyes. She's an academic all-star, spunky cheerleader, and talented actress with a kind heart and a ginormous personality. She's the happiest person alive, and if I could trade places with anyone on the planet, it would be her. Our son Parker, 14 at the time of my diagnosis, is absolutely dreamy. He's tall, fit, and gorgeous with mesmerizing green eyes and short dirty blonde hair. He's wicked smart with lightning-fast wit, but very reserved and quiet, so I basically hang on every word when he talks. He's a disciplined runner and, despite being an introvert, a skillful actor. Parker was born as my cuddly baby, so whether he likes it or not, I demand big hugs several times a day. His hugs tend to fix everything (almost). The Beans, as we call Ginger and Parker, are the kind of kids most parents could only dream of raising. I simply love them all the way, every day.

My furry best friend Piper is a mixture of yellow Labrador, Greyhound, princess, and linguistics expert. She is unusually obedient, has an extraordinary vocabulary, and will walk off-leash at my side, in cadence, whenever I want her to. While my neighbors' leashed dogs pull, yank, and bark at the sight of Piper, she just ignores them and politely walks along with me like a lady. Her discipline is incredible, as is her loyalty. Piper's quality of life is important to me, so I walked her several times daily, and chased her and her toys around our couch whenever she wanted me to. She was almost 10 years old at the time of my diagnosis and, as many stories go, she's the rescue pet that rescued me.

And finally, there's our duck, Handy. Yep. You read that correctly. DUCK! In November of 2018, we adopted a disabled Pekin duck from our friend's farm. The other ducks were being mean to Handy because her legs were twisted and she couldn't walk properly. My heart ached for her, so we brought her home. She became an incredible source of fun, love, and laughter in our house. Her big loud quacks made us giggle non-stop, as would watching her scoot around in a pullup diaper. We would take her on walks around our neighborhood in her red Radio Flyer wagon, go for adventure swims in our retention pond when it rained, and enjoy playtime on our big purple corduroy bean bag that she and Piper competed for. Handy's personality grew exponentially every day since she became a Koehler, and it lightened up our lives. She loved cuddling in my arms while being smothered with kisses and I loved being her mommy. Handy and Piper would become two of my greatest sources of comfort throughout this nightmare.

Professionally, I had created the career of my dreams and was enjoying every single ounce of my work. I do a few things, all of which allow me to focus on one thing: helping others live better and longer. Up first: I'm a fitness and sports performance expert with a master's degree in exercise and sport sciences from the University of Florida. I started teaching fitness at 15-years-old and, in the decades since, I've become more knowledgeable and passionate about making fitness understandable, attainable, and fun. While I used to love doing so, I haven't taught small classes in 20 years nor worked as a personal trainer in over a decade. Instead, I've laser-focused my efforts on opportunities that feed my desperate craving for mass impact. I don't want to help 50 people per day. I want to reach 500, 5,000, or 5 million. Most of my efforts are targeted toward teaching via mass media: through TV, radio, podcasts, books, magazines, online, and through large corporate speaking engagements or spokesperson contracts.

I always reference my role as a fitness expert first because it's at the core of who I am. However, one of the most extraordinary things that I do, and the thing you're going to read about the most, is race announcing. What is race announcing, you ask? Well, I announce or "host" the start and finish lines of running races. I usually work on a stage or tall tower, with my wireless microphone connected to a professional sound system. As runners and walkers arrive at the start line, exciting music plays while I engage, inform, and entertain. I tell them where to put their stuff, where to line up, share details about the course they're about to conquer, and plug sponsors. I also introduce dignitaries and singers, tell jokes, and recognize inspiring athletes. Everyone should feel welcomed, wanted, supported, and excited. If I've done my job well, they should all feel like they've become part of a team.

When all of that is done, I whip the crowd into a frenzy and then yell "go." Upon completion of each athlete's race, I await on a stage at the finish line making all sorts of happy noise, welcoming each of them in like a champion. My mission is to make every single person who crosses

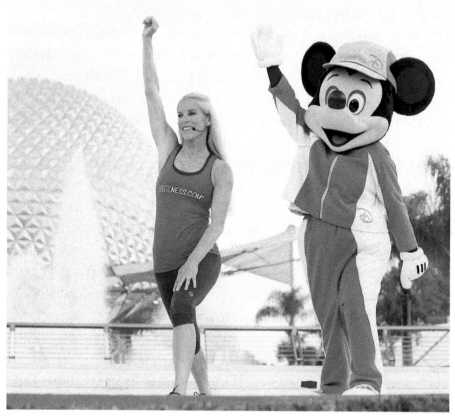

Teaching fitness at Disney's Epcot Center with Mickey Mouse.

the finish line feel like they've won the race, right down to the very last person. Technology allows me to congratulate most of these people by name, which they seem to get a royal kick out of. Most of my events have between 2,000 and 35,000 athletes participating so my role as the voice of the race is vital to its success. I provide structure and entertainment, and speak on behalf of each race organization as I lay praise on all of the participants. I pour a ton of energy and heart into announcing because I truly love and admire our runners. Think about it this way: as a fitness expert, I spend most of my time trying to convince people to exercise and eat wisely. But on race day, there is no need for arm-twisting or convincing. Instead, race organizers literally hand me thousands of people who have already decided exercising is a great idea. I'm simply asked to provide structure and show them a fabulous time. Ummm. Okay! I absolutely adore my events and athletes and take great pleasure and pride in my role. I've formed thousands of friendships through race announcing and this book almost serves as a love letter to the running industry. Some of my most harrowing days were made brighter because of it. This is where the words "dream career" come in.

Last, but definitely not least, I own one of the most successful and impactful school running programs in the USA and beyond. The Morning Mile™ is a before-school walking/running program that gives children the chance to start every day in an active way while enjoying fun, music, and friends. That's EVERY CHILD, EVERY DAY along with their families and school faculty, too. The program is supported by a wonderful system of rewards, which keeps students highly motivated and frequently congratulated. I created this program in the fall of 2010, and since then, it's been implemented at more than 400 schools in four different countries. My Morning Milers have run millions of miles, and endless amounts of children and families have adopted healthier lifestyles because of it. It is possibly the most important thing I have ever done professionally. My goal is to one day (soon) have The Morning Mile implemented at every school in America.

In short, I earn most of my income making happy noise and bossing people around. When it comes to being healthy, fit, and athletic, people seek out my opinion. And I give it to them with brutal honesty, quite often with a poke in the chest. That's why I'm called "bossy." My often loud and raucous work on a microphone is why I'm labeled "noisy." Most importantly, the only reason I get away with all of my bossiness and noisiness is because it comes wrapped in big love.

When I was home, I looked like a stay-at-home mom, shuttling kids to and from school and sports, cooking healthy meals, and encouraging family time. I would work on my computer, make calls, record podcasts, workout, and run errands while the kids were occupied, so I could be present once they were home. When I flew out for race weekends, Rob would hold down the fort and they all enjoyed eating pizza and ice cream, without me hovering.

The other most important thing to know is that I was incredibly healthy and uber-fit. I exercised aggressively, followed my own wise eating advice, and lived in a lean, hard, athletic body that I felt great about. I lifted a pretty impressive amount of weight for my size and was always in good enough shape to just pop into a half marathon and complete it without specifically training for it. Do I recommend that? Heck no! But do I recommend pursuing fitness so diligently and intelligently that you're always capable of running or walking 13.1 miles? Absolutely. Before my diagnosis, I would spend my workouts strength training in a variety of ways, walking, running, using an elliptical trainer, stretching a ton, and stand-up paddleboarding whenever possible. In fact, growing up in Florida made me a water sports junkie. Invite me to use your jet ski or drag me behind your boat for wakeboarding and we'll become instant friends. I've never smoked or used recreational drugs and I rarely drank alcohol. I walked the walk and was doing everything possible to be physically strong, promote my own health, and prevent disease. At the end of each chapter, I'll reveal my methods for staying fit throughout my treatment via monthly Fitzness Logs. It wasn't easy!

As a picture of health, I used to think that I was semi-immortal. But the truth is even super healthy people are vulnerable to disease. Despite being incredibly vibrant and strong at the time of my diagnosis, the cancer treatment obliterated me. Seriously, it made me feel like I was being dragged behind a horse for months at a time. But because of my incredible fitness at the start of my treatment, I was able to get up, dust myself off, and travel across the country doing the things I wanted to do. I was often sick as a dog while boarding those flights, but I refused to miss even one event on my calendar or one person at each race. No matter what, I showed up with my game face on and occasionally relied on a few miracles to get me through.

The misery inflicted by my cancer and treatment has been extreme, but I'm proud that while I was going through it, I was able to portray my experience as if it were a cakewalk. Why? In short, I'd rather people see me stand up instead of fall down. Complaining wouldn't have helped me because nobody could protect me from any of it. Sure, I had some help making life a bit easier. My family took great care of me, my friends brought meals and drove my kids around. Those things meant the world to me. However, I alone had to endure the cure. Sharing the pain and suffering while it was happening wouldn't have made any of it better and would have felt like a blatant request for pity. I wanted no part of that. I also had no interest in commiseration or unsolicited advice. I'm fortunate to have so many people who love and care for me, but I simply didn't want to be a beacon of sadness, sickness, or weakness. I've built an extraordinary career talking about being healthy and happy. Conversations about my suffering weren't going to make me or my audience any better. I also didn't want any of my race directors to have second thoughts about whether or not I was fit to do my job, so I got pretty good at convincing everyone that I was "fine."

I'm pretty confident that my stubbornness has been both my greatest and worst asset. I successfully announced over 20 races in nine different states during the most vicious rounds of chemo alone. I consider that proof that being a hardhead served me well. My other BFFs: determination and adrenaline. I'm 100% confident that if I'd had a regular day job during my treatment, I would have called in sick nonstop. But my passion for making happy noise for incredible people is so strong that I was compelled to show up no matter what. And once I was surrounded by thousands of amazing athletes, adrenaline became my go-go juice.

During my cancer nightmare, I wholeheartedly believe that my athletes gave me superpowers beyond what an average person could create on their own. Without them, there's no way I could have gone the distance. No way. I was also gifted with the most fabulous little pieces of kindness from tons of friends, and even plenty of strangers. Ok, so now you've got a good glimpse at who I am, and what my life was like BEFORE everything changed. Before C-Day.

December 28, 2018. Friday.

As I've done many times before, I went in for my annual mammogram and walked out, celebrating a clean bill of health. While some folks avoid or ignore all sorts of annual exams, I've been committed to mine for years. With mammograms, specifically, I started getting them yearly after I gave birth to my daughter, Ginger, in 2003. About a week after her delivery, I found a lump in my right breast. I was nursing, thus touching my boobs a bunch, and it wasn't hard to find. I remember it feeling like a popcorn kernel. After a quick appointment with my obstetrician, I was referred for a mammogram and ultrasound. A mammogram involves placing your breast between two plates and using X-ray imaging to discover suspicious findings. It provides images of your entire breast. Ultrasound is an imaging method that uses high-frequency sound waves to produce images of structures within your body. It is a far more personal experience, with a technician or radiologist manually capturing the images while rubbing a handheld transducer over your body. It is better at distinguishing between benign fluid-filled cysts and solid masses. With Ginger in her infant carrier on the table with me as the ultrasound tech did her thing, all I could think was, "Cut them off!! Cut them both off! Just please just let me spend forever here with this baby." Thankfully, I was told my popcorn kernel was just some sort of calcification from nursing, and I was fine. Phew! I've never been so grateful in my life.

One of the valuable things I learned back then was that through my insurance, annual mammograms were free. So, while so many women were intentionally avoiding them because "they hurt" (no, they don't), or they wanted to avoid any potential bad news, I took the opposite position. While mammograms weren't fun, they really only caused me slight discomfort, and financially … they didn't cost me anything. If I were ever to have some sort of cancerous jerk growing inside me, I would want to know about it and start killing it as soon as possible. Since that day, I haven't missed one single annual mammogram. Nor have I missed a yearly skin check, pap smear, dental exam … you name it! As well, I've been an avid promoter of annual and self-exams to my large audiences as a fitness expert. I've spent tons of time on national and local news outlets, radio, podcasts, online/live presentations advocating for the prioritization of early detection.

Moving on. I left this mammogram, thrilled with a letter confirming no trouble in my mammaries. When I got into my car, I took some time to post on Instagram (@Fitzness), my annual reminder for everyone else to go get their stuff squeezed. Sadly, this clean bill of health would not immunize me from trouble moving forward.

Chapter 2

I'm Definitely Dying

February 21, 2019. Thursday.

Less than two months after my mammogram, my whole world was turned upside down. While standing naked in my hotel bathroom at Disney World, I casually used my right hand to scratch the underboob on my left side (yes, underboob - I've always called it that, and you know exactly what I'm referring to). Mid scratch, I felt something that felt like a bean. Something that definitely did not belong there. There was no confusion. There was no wondering whether or not it was dense breast tissue. It was a bean that should not have been. Since I had my cell phone in the bathroom with me, I instantly picked it up and called my gynecologist. I didn't hem and haw about it. I didn't check with a friend to ask for advice about what I should do. I picked up my phone and contacted my doctor immediately. Honestly, I wish more people would do the same. Addressing symptoms swiftly is often the difference between life and death. Within about two minutes from finding the bean, I had an appointment booked for the following Monday. I was taking it seriously, and so were they. Now my challenge was to try and forget about my bean for the weekend. I was there to run the Disney Princess 10K, and support my runners who were also taking part. I didn't tell anyone, as I specifically do not enjoy drama. My gut told me that I definitely had breast cancer, but there was a slim chance my bean would be something benign like it had been 16 years earlier. I have a stringent policy of not crying over milk that hasn't spilled yet, so I was pretty successful with my efforts to relax and enjoy.

Instead of agonizing over my mystery bean, I swam in the resort pool and dined with friends. I also completed the 10K on Friday morning. I had planned to run the race, but since some old kickboxing injuries were acting up (yes, I used to fight competitively), I chose to just walk it with my friends Demarie Bottai and Sean Matlock. It was such a delightful experience. While I usually savor challenging myself by actually running races, sometimes it's okay to do the complete opposite. The weather was beautiful, clear, in the high 60s, and we had an absolute blast walking and talking for 6.2 miles. Nothing hurt, I never felt taxed, and the whole experience boiled down to refreshing active fun. The next day, I did my part to support those running the half marathon. This has become a bit of a tradition when I'm at a Disney race weekend. If I'm not running a race, I usually have a pretty sweet spot in a VIP tent that sits right up against the chute (the road leading up to the finish line). I wait there to cheer on my runners, and most of them stop by to share sweaty hugs before they complete their race. My runners: people who I've helped prepare in some way for their races, people whom I've met through race announcing, and those who eventually became friends. I love them all, and they seem to love me back. I'm invested in their success, so when they reach me near the end of their race, they're congratulated by someone they know cares about them deeply.

February 25. Monday.

I casually checked in for my 1:20 p.m. visit with the physician assistant at my gynecologist's office. While doing a manual exam, she easily felt my lump at "4 o'clock" and stated that she didn't think it would be anything serious. However, she was still going to refer me on for imaging. Although I would have insisted on imaging anyway, I was happy to hear she didn't think my lump was going to be lethal. I wasn't panicked (yet, anyway), but her lack of alarm was helpful to my psyche. I already believed that I had breast cancer, but without a doctor's confirmation, agonizing over it would be a waste of my energy. I was able to schedule a mammogram and ultrasound for Thursday morning and, once again, didn't feel pressure to notify my family. I did, however, decide to tell my friend Cheryl Tyrone about my lump. I visited her husband's office for a facial that week and confided in her because she was treated for breast cancer in 2017 and beat it. I'm so glad I did because she would become a huge source of guidance and comfort for me as things played out.

February 28. Thursday.

The morning rolled in and I nonchalantly headed out for imaging with the radiologist I'd been seeing for 16 years, Dr. Judith Yancey. Things got rolling with a mammogram, and then I was escorted into a little room for my ultrasound. As I laid on the table while the ultrasound tech smeared goo on my boob and started ultrasound-ing me (yes, that's a verb), I was able to see the screen she was looking at. My tech was poker-faced and, since she's not a doctor, she wasn't really allowed to say anything about what she saw. But as she went over my lump, I could see it. A weird little black oval with a white border. It could be a benign cyst, right? I still wasn't panicking.

After we finished, Dr. Yancey came in, acting a little odd, a little jumpier, and more breathless than usual. My "spidey senses" were definitely tingling. She sat on the chair in front of the screen, squeezed some more warm goo on my boob, and started ultrasound-ing. Once again, that jerky little lump appeared, which is when she said, "That lump looks suspicious." I still wasn't panicking. But then she said the words that left zero doubt in my mind that I had cancer. "You also have a few hard swollen lymph nodes that I'm concerned about." PANIC! At that point, wet stuff started shooting out of my eyes and I knew I was in big trouble. One lump — not too bad. Maybe a little surgery could fix it. A lump and some lymph nodes? I knew in my heart that I was doomed for surgery, chemotherapy, radiation, and possibly even an early demise. I was absolutely terrified. As I sat there sobbing, they told me they were going to quickly share the news with my gyno so that she could refer me to a surgeon who could order a biopsy. Ugh. I already knew what was going on! I had breast cancer. Life was about to change, drastically. And I could be on track to die young.

Now, I can honestly tell you, and most folks would agree, I'm the ultimate optimist. Doom and gloom annoy the crap out of me, even when they're fairly justified. But as I walked out to my car, all I could think about were Ginger and Parker and how much of their beautiful lives I was going to miss out on. I couldn't get past the fact that my story was going to be the perfect tale of tragedy. The fitness expert who did almost everything right health-wise, while working so diligently to help others live long and well was going to be killed by cancer at a young age. Oh, the irony! I did not want to be the perfect tragic tale. But yeah. I was definitely going to die.

After sobbing in my car for half an hour, I walked over to Cheryl Tyrone's office, who conveniently happened to be right next door to Dr. Yancey's. Cheryl is the sweetest. A lovely person in any situation, but she really comforted me that day as I boohooed at her desk. She shared a bit

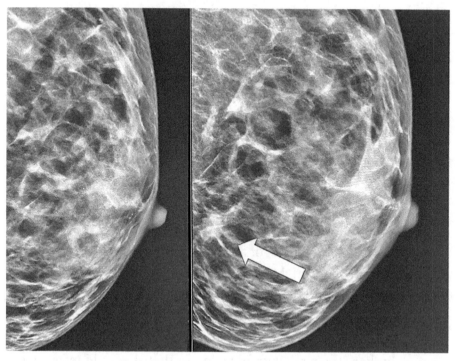

Clean Mammogram. 12/27/18   14 MM Tumor on Mammogram. 2/28/19

more about her personal experience beating breast cancer and then did the most helpful and important thing of all. She told me about her medical team, which consisted of three specialty doctors here in Gainesville. These three are considered by many to be the "Dream Team." It consisted of Dr. Lucio Gordan (Hematology-Oncology), who is the President of all Florida Cancer Specialists and Research Institutes (FCS), Dr. Cherylle Hayes (Radiology-Oncology) who is Medical Director of The Cancer Center of North Florida Regional Healthcare (TCC), and Dr. Panagiotis "Peter" Sarantos, a top-notch surgeon who specializes in, you guessed it, breast cancer.

When I left Cheryl's, I spoke with my gyno's office, and they promised to send a referral over to Dr. Sarantos for me. They thought I would be able to see him in a week, *maybe*. Nope. Wrong. Instead, I got to see Dr. Sarantos that same day at 1 p.m. Thankfully, he didn't mess around with cancer and was happy to squeeze me into his schedule right away. In the meantime, I had to tell Rob what was going on. That wasn't a fun call to make. I tried to act casual, "Hey, can you meet for lunch?" He agreed and we met at a little restaurant called Bolay. Rob was on duty and showed up in his police uniform. He could tell that something was wrong immediately. I told him about finding the lump and about all of the appointments I'd secretly had that week. He hugged me tight and told me that it was going to be okay, and that he would be with me every inch of the way. I believed the part about him being there, but how could anyone know *if* I would be okay? I sat at our table and cried a bunch while he, a bit shell-shocked, absorbed the information. And then, we made a pact to do whatever it would take to beat whatever I was dealing with. We went through the motions and ordered food, but I don't recall either of us eating much of it.

When we arrived at Dr. Sarantos' office an hour or so later, I was pretty anxious. Dr. Sarantos was smart, soft-spoken, and compassionate. As an aside, he has a Greek background, and all of the ladies in town go crazy for him. It's like having Elvis as your surgeon. He's got the wavy black hair and fans far and wide. Mention Dr. Sarantos to any woman in Gainesville, and she will practically pass out with the swoon! When he entered my exam room, he performed a manual exam of my lump and nodes and then explained my options for biopsies. He wanted to provide me with the quickest and least invasive option, which sounded great. We decided on a punch biopsy, and magically, we were able to schedule it for 7:30 a.m. the next day. I was pleased that my waiting and wondering were going to be kept to a minimum. He also told me that while he couldn't make any diagnosis without the biopsy, the irregular borders of my lump were quite concerning. Ouch! It was more proof that I had what I already knew deep down that I had. Stressed to the max, I did quite a bit of crying while talking with him. I told him about Ginger and Parker and how I couldn't leave them too early. He gently held my hands, looked into my eyes, and assured me that I was going to be okay.

I headed home that afternoon with intentions of not freaking out until I had official results, but that was hard to do. I was also determined not to scare my kids until I had actual reason to. Ginger and Parker did not need to worry about this unnecessarily. However, my 78-year-old mother just so happened to be arriving that day for a weekend visit. Ugh. I would have liked to save her some anxiety, but since I'd be having that biopsy the next morning, I really didn't have a choice but to fill her in. Once she had arrived and settled in, I gave her the scoop. Clearly, that's not the kind of news any mother likes to receive, so I tried to convince her it would be nothing, even though I wasn't convinced of that myself. To this day I'm still not sure if she believed me.

Fitzness Log

At this point, I was still working out at full volume. Because of my new stressors, I might have even been putting in a little more time and effort than usual. I worked out five or six days a week at my incredible local gym, Gainesville Health and Fitness Center (GHFC). Each workout would last an hour or two and I'd do any combination of running, walking, using the elliptical trainer, stretching, and strength training. While challenging my already-fit body was a high priority, I was also relying on exercise to exhaust the anxiety accruing in my mind. I love weight training so much that I've often referred to dumbbells as my "boyfriends." Those boyfriends of mine got lots of attention this month.

Chapter 3

Nostril Wigs and Hot Pants

March 1. Friday.

I cried in my kitchen as I prepared to leave the house for my biopsy. Folks, I can assure you that I am not, or better yet was not, a big crier. Cancer changed all of that. Crying in the kitchen became one of my things. In fact, I also became really great at crying in my car, bathroom, bedroom, and backyard. Hotels? Yep! I can blubber out of town as well. If you need someone to cry at your next event, I may be available. My mom asked if I was okay, and I told her I was just stressed. That was the truth. I had always managed anxiety with optimism and rationalism, so it rarely affected me. But the pressure that comes with cancer is like no other and my magical stress management powers had been rendered useless.

Upon arrival, I was brought into a dark little room, where I changed into a gown, laid on the table, and waited. Dr. Jani entered, introduced himself, and smeared warm goo on my left breast. The deal here was that he was going to find my lump under ultrasound and use the guidance of the TV screen to poke his big fat needles straight into my lump and swollen lymph nodes. Once he entered the targeted areas with each needle, he would hit a trigger, and the needle would grab a chunk of the target and remove it to be sent off for testing. He would also leave tiny little metal clips inside the tumor and nodes so they could be easily identified in the future. He started by injecting lidocaine into my armpit and breast, which was not a lot of fun. Can you imagine someone sticking multiple needles into your armpit or your boob? It was a bizarre experience. Once these areas were numb, it was time for him to use the pencil-sized needles (mild exaggeration) for the actual biopsies. I was warned I would feel "pressure," which would apply if you describe "pressure" the same way you would describe being shot with a .22 caliber rifle at close range. As he worked and I felt more than just "pressure," I let loose with a plethora of my favorite curse words. And, since I could see the screen he was utilizing, I was able to watch as those needles went through me. It was more than freaky. Did I mention that I'm squeamish? Oh yes, I'm a total medical wimp. And that didn't help at all. He drove those fat needles into me and, when I verbally agreed that I was ready for him to do his thing, POW! He pulled the trigger and grabbed some tissue. The first few times he did it were uncomfortable. The last four were punishing. If he tried it again, I may have deployed Rob to disarm him and create a diversion so I could shimmy out the window. I was confident that I was going to be sore for a while. And I was. The whole process took about an hour, and I was given an ice pack for the pain. I was then sent into another room for yet another mammogram.

While I was waiting for the mammogram, an old friend of mine, Dr. Jill Wolkstein, who's also a radiologist, stopped by to check on me. At some point during our conversation, I expressed confusion about having a clean mammogram less than seven weeks prior. How could it happen so quickly? Her response was, "Well, it has to start sometime." That made sense. Think about it. Most people think that once a clear scan has arrived, we're arbitrarily safe for a year or close to it. But who's to say that the day or even the second after an exam is complete, a cell doesn't start going rogue and become cancerous? I've recently met several other women who've found lumps almost immediately after having mammograms. In fact, I was just told about a neighbor who found a lump SIX DAYS post-mammogram. Crazy, right? This makes the best case for self-exams. If I hadn't found my lump and it had gone untreated until my next mammogram, I'd surely be a goner.

The aftermath of the punch biopsy was about as fun as the biopsy itself. My left breast and armpit were completely black and blue, and I was pretty darn sore for a while. In the grand scheme of things this wasn't such a big deal, but it really did hurt! In fact, while walking around over the next week, I had to keep my left hand in my pocket or tucked into my shorts to minimize movement.

Although you're going to hear a bit about my cursing here, I want you to know that I'm not actually a potty mouth. Unsurprisingly, cancer has warranted a bit of foul language. Sorry, mom!

March 5th. Tuesday.

I got the call. I was sitting in my bedroom around 5 p.m. preparing to take Ginger out for a college consulting appointment when Dr. Sarantos rang me up. He was sorry to tell me that my biopsy results were positive and that I did, indeed, have breast cancer. Specifically, I had invasive ductal carcinoma, stage 2B. He said that they'd know more when the genetic testing on my tissue samples was complete, but for now I had the big C and he was referring me to hematology-oncologist Dr. Lucio Gordan. Surprisingly, this didn't leave me in a blubbering ball of tears, because I already *knew* I had cancer. Once again Dr. Sarantos tried to assure me that I would be treatable. Did I believe him? Not necessarily. I figured that he probably always tried to stay positive for his patients. At least at the beginning, right? I didn't know. Perhaps he was just blowing smoke to prevent me from melting down. But I would have to wait and see to know for sure.

After receiving my results, I called Rob at work. He assured me that I was going to be okay and told me how much he loved me. Although this was devastating news, I had some important momming to do, so I put on a smile, threw my beautiful daughter in the car, and headed out to our meeting like nothing was wrong. I remember putting Queen's "Bohemian Rhapsody" on for us to sing to and take my mind off things.

31

Sadly, it didn't work. She had no idea what I was going through and resisted my fun song, opting for a slow one instead. The sad tune felt like the theme song for all of the horrible thoughts swirling around in my head. Rob joined us for the college consult and we got through the hour-long appointment passing weird looks at each other. We talked about Ginger's grades, scores, classes, leadership opportunities and more, all while I was trying to process the future or my potential lack of it.

While being diagnosed with any type of cancer is terrifying, mine was particularly scary for one gargantuan reason: It was very aggressive and traveling at warp speed. Less than seven weeks prior, my mammogram was completely clean. Now, I already had a 14 mm tumor, at least three infected lymph nodes, and possibly more. This cancer was on the go and hell-bent on taking me out. I was desperately hoping it hadn't already made its way into my liver, lungs, or brain.

March 6. Wednesday.

I was scheduled to meet with Dr. Gordan at 3 p.m., but woke up to a phone call from my new radiology oncologist, Dr. Cherylle Hayes. She knew that I had an appointment with Dr. Gordan that afternoon and, since they're in the same building, she was hoping I would stop by her office a few minutes prior to get a little face time together. I was happy to do so and really appreciated the personal outreach. It certainly meant a lot to me as a freaked-out new cancer patient to have that call and invitation come in. As instructed, I stopped by her office for the intro, and her nurses brought me into an exam room to wait. After a few minutes, Dr. Hayes made her appearance. She sauntered in wearing scrubs, a puffy leopard-print winter vest, and high heels. She was absolutely gorgeous and had tremendous swagger. In fact, she was crazy cocky and I loved it. I'm completely attracted to power and confidence, and Dr. Hayes oozed both. She's revered as an aggressive innovator in radiology who's highly effective at what she does. Both her mother and sister had breast cancer (her sister died because of it), so she has a personal vendetta against my disease, which I really enjoy. She was charismatic, kind, and enthusiastically reassuring that we were going to kill that cancer of mine. She instructed me to make an appointment when I was ready to move forward with radiation.

I soon walked next-door to the hematology side of the building to meet Dr. Gordan, but before he arrived, Rob and I spent some time with his nurse, Tracey Curtis, APRN. She was very warm and her duty was to give us a crash course on breast cancer and all of the treatment options for it. This took about an hour and, while very helpful, she went into explicit detail about all sorts of possibilities (mostly horrible) that I didn't necessarily need to know. Most of it was relevant, but some of the scary stuff was not in my future and just added to my stress. Let me be clear. There are no fun highlights involved in cancer treatments. Sure, killing cancer is awesome and so is remission, but the process of getting there is harsh. I was given the scoop on treatment plans for all stages and types of breast cancer, including those with a genetic component. Some of the groovy experiences I may or may not have to face included extreme sickness, complete mastectomy, hysterectomy, hair loss, anemia, infection, radiation burns, and spontaneous combustion. The last one is a lie, but you get my drift. The list was long and ugly. In hindsight, I wish we had waited until we knew the specifics of my particular disease to go over all of the possibilities, so she could have saved me from some of the horror stories.

Dazed and confused, I finally got to meet Dr. Gordan who had a reputation for being a world-class cancer killer. Besides being ridiculously bright and experienced, he was kind, calm, patient, and super handsome. All three of my doctors could save lives *and* win beauty pageants. Fun! During the appointment I was told that I would do chemo before surgery and radiation, but that I wouldn't know exactly what chemotherapy drugs I would receive, nor how often I would get them until they got my pathology reports back. Many people have asked me why I didn't do surgery first, and I can share that my first instinct about it all was, "Cut this crap out of me, now!" But the reason chemo would come first was because once cancer travels to the lymph nodes, there is the potential for cancer cells to start spreading through the rest of the body via the lymphatic system. That would have given those speedy little cancer cells plenty of time to travel about wreaking havoc elsewhere. By starting chemotherapy first, they were systematically treating my entire body by shrinking or killing any cancer cells no matter where they were. Once they had done that, I would then undergo surgery to remove whatever cancer was left, and lastly get radiation therapy.

One of the things I really appreciate about Dr. Gordan is how thorough he was. I often showed up with little lists, so I wouldn't forget to address my concerns when we were in the room together. I'm pretty confident that if I'd had 43 hours' worth of questions, he would have stuck around and answered them all. And he always considered Rob and asked him if he had any questions as well. I can't imagine going through this with a physician who made me feel rushed or unimportant. All three of my doctors worked to make me feel like I was the most important patient in the world. Besides talking about treatment options, I did a lot of crying on that first day. I was terrified of dying and so fearful of leaving my kids, Rob, and all of the other amazing people in my life. When I asked Dr. Gordan whether or not he thought we could beat my cancer, he said, "Absolutely! Your cancer is very treatable. We should have no problems." That was exactly what I needed to hear. His confidence was calming and reassuring, and I was able to stop imagining my own funeral.

In light of both the bad and good news, it was going to be a hard night. I hadn't told my kids about any of this yet because I didn't want to freak them out prematurely, but it was officially time to do so. After meeting with my two oncologists, I had enough information to speak honestly and confidently about my situation. I chose to tell them separately. Parker is a quiet and thoughtful kid who deals with private conversations best. Ginger has a big bubbly personality with a huge heart to match, but she also grieves in a very big way. I wanted to allow each of them the opportunity to receive the information and ask questions without any interference from the other. I chose to tell Parker first since he would most likely handle the situation quietly. After dinner, when Ginger went into our home gym to exercise, Rob and I brought Parker into his room to talk. I took the "bad news, good news" approach. I told him that I found a lump a couple of weeks back, had gone through some tests, and unfortunately, I had breast cancer. I reassured him that I caught it fairly early and that my doctors were absolutely confident I was going to be fine. I told him I would feel kind of bad and look kind of weird for a while, but I was going to be okay. As expected, he processed things quietly and asked a few simple questions. The main thing I remember him telling me was, "Mommy, I think you're going to look cute bald!" Swoon. Total swoon. I'm so lucky to have a sweet boy who loves me so much. His calm and caring comfort made this conversation go as smoothly as possible. Now, many months later, I asked Parker if he ever thought I was going to die. "Definitely," he said. Yikes! I thought I'd done such a great job convincing him I'd be okay, but apparently he had doubts anyway. When I asked him why he never spoke to me about that, he simply stated that he didn't want to make things more difficult for me. Poor thing.

Here's one of the reasons I had to plan out and execute my conversations with Ginger and Parker precisely: we had recently lost our good friend, Charlene Molloy, 51, to pancreatic cancer. She was the gorgeous, vibrant, and adoring mother of one of their soccer teammates, Garrett, and his older sister, Marissa. I coached Ginger, Parker, Garrett, and our talented Rabid Alien soccer team for many years. Over time, our team became like a family. Charlene and her husband, Glenn, were very dedicated parents who cheered hard from the sidelines and made me laugh with sarcastic comments as I paced in front of them. Losing my sparkly friend was incredibly hard. It was painful to see her family suffer and horrible to know she was fighting a losing battle. If you're unfamiliar, the five-year survival rate for pancreatic cancer is 9%; it's devastating. After her diagnosis, I spent lots of time with Charlene. I helped her stay fit, drove her to the occasional appointment, and even picked up Garrett from school on occasion. Parker joined me to take Charlene to radiation once and he was so very compassionate toward her. Her weakness was obvious and I was proud that he handled her with care. Our lives had become fairly intertwined with the Molloys and we simply carried this whole family in our hearts daily. After she passed, the four of us went to her funeral, and it was an agonizing experience for everyone. Fast forward to my diagnosis, I was nervous that my kids would instantly identify her cancer with mine. The thought of losing a parent while you're still a child probably seems pretty outlandish until you witness it happening up close and personal as they had.

While I couldn't really guarantee my survival, the odds with breast cancer are almost 90% better than those with pancreatic cancer. Convincing the kids that not all cancers were created equal was vital to relay in a compelling and believable way. In fact, Charlene remained on my mind throughout this battle, especially during the early months. As always, perspective commanded my behavior, and while I would sit sobbing in an exam room feeling endless amounts of fear, I would often imagine how much more difficult things must have been for her with a far more vicious diagnosis. It didn't always stop my tears, but it made me grateful to be facing better odds. I wish all cancers were as well-funded, well-researched, easily identifiable, and curable as breast cancer is.

I'm not suggesting that all cancers aren't scary. Trust me. I truly believe they are and can attest that mine was devastating. If you've never heard the words "you have cancer," good for you! But I have a hunch that 100% of you have had your world rocked by learning that someone you cared about was diagnosed. The first thing we associate with cancer is death. We think, "Please don't let this person die!" Or in my case, "Please don't let this kill me." It's all pretty dreadful. However, thanks to generous people and organizations who fund research, those ingenious scientists who do the research and those caring medical professionals who implement it, many cancers are now curable. Many, but not all. Breast cancer cure rates are upwards of 93%, but the death rates are still far too high considering one in eight women in America is diagnosed with it. The prevalence is more than disturbing, but I hope that science will continue to improve cure rates and maybe even find some sort of vaccination or prevention tool.

While my cancer invaded my boob with bad intentions, I was able to increase my odds of survival by discovering that evil tumor within just a few weeks of its genesis. It's alarming to think about what would have happened had I not rubbed my underboob and found that tumor. If it had not been discovered until my next scheduled mammogram 10 months later, I'm 100% confident that every organ in my body would have been riddled with disease at that point. My cancer was spreading swiftly and aggressively. Had I not squeezed my stuff, I'd likely not be sitting here today writing this noisy comeback story.

After we spoke with Parker, I braced myself to tell Ginger. When she came out of the gym, Rob and I sat her down on the living room couch and gave her a similar explanation. Bad news, good news. My poor sweet girl just sobbed inconsolably. It was heart-breaking. No matter what we said to comfort her, she just wailed. I can't blame her. I would have responded the same exact way had it been my mom. In fact, I remember bawling my eyes out because my mom had to have back surgery when I was a kid. Cancer would have been inordinately more difficult to bear. We did lots of hugging, crying, and talking, but I think it took a solid hour to calm her down. I often gush about the way Ginger beams with joy. On the flip side, when the happiest person alive is heartbroken it's excruciating to witness. Eventually we were able to calm her down and I hoped that I was able to convince her that I wasn't going to die anytime soon. Ginger continued to struggle emotionally for quite a while. Parenting with cancer is interesting. As I was struggling to convince myself that I would be okay, as a mom I was simultaneously declaring my guaranteed curability. We'll do, or say, anything to fix things for them, won't we?

As I discuss visiting "the cancer center" throughout these pages, I'd like to help you visualize the place. All of my oncology visits for chemotherapy and radiation took place in one giant building. The right side of the building was occupied by Dr. Gordon's crew at the Florida Cancer Specialists and Research Institute. This is where I went for chemo. The left side of the building is where Dr. Hayes reigned as the queen of radiation of The Cancer Center at North Florida. All of my zapping took place on that side. Ninety percent of my medical appointments took place in this building, which contains one massive lobby that both sides share. You'll hear about it a lot, so I think it's helpful to know this.

March 7. Thursday.

While meeting with my interns at one of my favorite local restaurants, The Bagel Bakery, I got a call from Dr. Gordan's nurse, Tracey Curtis. She told me that my cancer was referred to as "double positive." It was HER2 positive, estrogen receptor-positive, and progesterone receptor-negative. While she went through the list of things I was positive for, all I could think of was "Fuck! Did I have to be positive for EVERYTHING? I'm definitely going to die." In fact, I'm pretty sure I said that to her. She responded with "No, no, no. In this case, the 'positives' are usually a good thing because it means we have identified the type of trigger for the type of cancer we're dealing with and we know how to kill it." Oh, okay — I guess that sounded like a good deal. One of the things I was positive for, HER2, is the type of cancer that grows rapidly. It's aggressive. Hence, a lump and three lymph nodes turning up cancerous within less than two months. However, she said that the type of cancer that grows really fast usually dies really fast as well. That was music to my ears.

Then she explained exactly what type of chemotherapy I was going to have. It was a protocol that included four different chemo drugs. Taxotere, Carboplatin, Perjeta, and Herceptin. I'd have these four drugs on Mondays, every three weeks, for six rounds. We eventually referred to these four drugs as "mean chemo." When that was over, I'd continue on with Herceptin-only (this would eventually change) every three weeks for eight more rounds. I'd also have surgery once I completed the first six rounds of the mean stuff to remove whatever was left of my tumor and infected nodes. And finally radiation soon after that. I was in for a lot of fun. Oh! And, my long golden blonde hair was almost definitely going to fall out. Greaaaat.

One looming unanswered question was whether or not I would need a full mastectomy — the complete removal of one or both breasts. While I wasn't as panicked about replacing my natural boobs for falsies, I was definitely concerned about having to endure such a "big deal" surgery. Yes, they're "just boobs," but removing any body part involves plenty of pain, trauma, healing time, and emotional strain. Also, rarely is a mastectomy just one single surgery. Quite often, women end up with more operations on the road to reconstruction. I was ready to do whatever it took to save my life, but I was desperately hoping a full mastectomy was not in my future. I know many women do it because it's mandated, while many do it out of fear. But I'm a science girl and chose to work with statistics. If there was no statistical benefit to having the full deal, I would be elated to skip it. I would have my answer once the blood we'd sent out for genetic testing returned.

In 2013, actress Angelina Jolie made the BRCA1 gene famous when she underwent a preventative mastectomy. Her mother, Marcheline Bertrand, died at the young age of 56 after battling both breast and ovarian cancers. Bertrand's mother (ovarian) and sister (breast) also died of cancer. Being BRCA1 positive gave Jolie reasonable confidence that she would also face the beast if she didn't take preemptive measures. Eventually, Jolie also had a salpingo-oophorectomy, which is an ovary and fallopian tube removal. Honestly, a new cancer diagnosis was awful on its own. Knowing that I might have a genetic predisposition for it and could have possibly passed it along to Ginger was definitely haunting. If I did have that predisposition, it looked like many surgeries would probably be in both of our futures.

Back to my lunch meeting with my fabulous interns. I work closely with my alma mater, the University of Florida. Every semester I give a presentation to a group of graduating seniors in the College of Health and Human Performance, where I earned my Master of Exercise and Sport Sciences degree. And every semester I also host one to five full-time interns. At this point, I had a smarty pants trio of ladies: Emily, Audrey, and Lexi. That day I was meeting with Emily and Lexi. Knowing that things were going to change for me very quickly and that there was one month of the internship remaining, I had to tell them what was going on. I didn't like doing so, but I sugar-coated everything, so they wouldn't worry. I try not to cross-contaminate business and personal stuff too much, but I really didn't have much of a choice. I warned them that they may need to be a little more independent moving forward, but I knew that they were capable of that.

When I left The Bagel Bakery, I headed home to do something that I knew I couldn't put off. See, while I'm fairly bold about sharing details about my profession and my pets, I normally keep my personal life private. I've often felt a bit put off by folks sharing all sorts of personal details, especially hardships, on social media. Some people love to divulge everything, particularly the miserable stuff. Good for them, but it's not for me. I'm a happy girl who promotes health and I just don't want any part of the other side of things. I'm not suggesting that real life doesn't have its downsides, but blatant requests for pity and the airing of dirty laundry is really unappealing. I desperately wanted to keep my breast cancer diagnosis quiet and figure things out in secret as I went. But my impending baldness meant that wouldn't be possible. I knew for sure that the second I stepped on a stage bald or with a wig, people were going to start asking questions. What I decided to do was release a video message on social media to share the basics of what I knew. In the meantime, I had been aggressively contacting my family members and closest friends so none of them had to find out through the grapevine.

The other people I was zealously contacting were my race directors. These are the people that organize the running events I announce. My race calendar for the year was jam-packed with extraordinary events that I had zero intentions of missing. I was convinced that my announcing schedule was the best in the nation, and I wasn't giving up even one of the career opportunities that I rightfully earned and loved so much. But first, I had to contact these wonderful bosses of mine to let them know what was going on. I'm an independent contractor for each, so I had lots of phone calls to make. Fortunately for me, my race directors are some of the best humans on the planet and I truly feel a quality friendship with them all. It was hard to deliver my news over and over, but my message remained constant: "I've been diagnosed with breast cancer. It's an awful situation, but I'm curable. I'm going to be treated aggressively but I am NOT going to miss your race. I will be there, and I will perform as expected." I tried to make most of these calls via FaceTime as I have a pretty strong policy that tough talks should be had in person and face to face whenever possible. Time and time again I was greeted with sorrow, followed by faith. Every last one of my race directors were pained that I'd be going through something so difficult, but they all told me that they were 100% with me. If I was healthy enough for announcing, they wanted me at their events. They also told me that if at any point before race day I had to tap out, they'd totally understand. How could I ask for more? These were hard calls to make, but I put on my biggest smile as I made them so no one had any reason to doubt me.

Sitting at my kitchen table, I crafted a little outline and then hit record on my phone to create my "I have breast cancer" video. I revealed my basic diagnosis of breast cancer, that I'd have chemo, surgery, radiation, and most importantly that my doctors had assured me a cure. I said that I'd continue announcing my races, growing The Morning Mile, and promoting Fitzness. I requested zero pity or unsolicited advice, but let folks know that they could root for me and send warm wishes. My video ended up being about five minutes long, and I assure you it's the weirdest five minutes of footage I've ever recorded. I've been on camera for television and online productions since I was about 20 years old and this was the definitive lowlight. It's still available on my Fitzness page on Facebook and on my YouTube channel. It's a weird moment in my history. Go watch it if you'd like. I've spent my career talking about you, you, and you. Almost every second of footage recorded has always been to make fitness and sport more understandable, attainable, and fun. Talking about me … in this way … was not a comfortable thing to do. I recorded a few takes and chose the one I felt was the least uncomfortable for publishing. I decided to wait until I'd contacted everyone on my shortlist before I shared the video publicly.

Next up on this very long day was an MRI (magnetic resonance imaging) scan, which would take detailed images of the organs and tissues in my body. This, in addition to an echocardiogram, was required before I would be allowed to start chemo on Monday. Everything had been scheduled quite urgently and quickly, so I was squeezed into a 5 p.m. appointment at the end of the day. While many people can handle this mostly non-invasive procedure with ease, I am incredibly claustrophobic and found it to be one of the most disturbing experiences of my life. Generally MRIs require people to lie down on a thin bed, facing up while they are slid into a long narrow metal tube that has fancy X-Ray technology around it. You literally just lie there.

My first surprise came when I arrived and was told I would have an IV placed in my right arm so they could inject some sort of nuclear fluid into me. Halfway through my 40-minute imaging session, the dye would be injected in order to make my cancer more visible. Did I mention that I also have a legit phobia of needles? The tears started pouring as soon as the MRI lady sat me down for the IV. She seemed very nice at this point and made an effort to comfort me, which I appreciated. Once she successfully inserted the IV, she sent me into a dressing room to change into a fancy hospital gown, after which I was brought into the imaging room.

My second surprise came when I was told I would not be lying on my back, like normal. Instead, I was going to be lying face down in a Superman position — With my arms over my head and my face in a crappy little face cradle, similar to that of a massage table, only worse. Once I assumed the position, they would proceed to clamp each of my boobs with metal plates, pinning them, and me, into place. I was completely unprepared for this, but when she told me to climb up and lie down, I did. I didn't even take a moment to take a deep breath. I just climbed up and went face down as I was instructed to do. The second I laid down, she told me, "If you move at all, everything will be ruined."

I was given no time to adjust. No suggestion to pull my hair back. Nothing. And as I laid down, I instantly became uncomfortable and my anxiety started to amplify. It's amazing what happens when someone tells me to be still. I become acutely aware of everything that is wrong with me at the moment. My body was in a bizarre position. My nose itched. My eyes twitched. I felt every millimeter of myself, especially the things that weren't perfect. I needed to crack my back. My hair was all over my face. I was already very uncomfortable. One by one, she clamped on to each of my breasts with those plates, imprisoning my body and my mind. Can you imagine being pinned down by the boobs? It was something straight out of medieval times. Guys, perhaps you could relate by imagining being pinned face-down, and held into place by your junk and nose? Then she put big padded earphones over my ears, which made me feel like my whole head was being covered with a pillow. I told her I didn't want to wear them, but since MRI machines are loud and have a constant banging noise, I risked hearing damage if I did not comply. I tried to stay calm. I tried really hard. But once she had me clamped down into that awful position, with my head smothered, and then slid me into that tube, I completely freaked out. And not just a little freak-out. I had a 5-star crying, screaming kind of freak-out. I felt like I had been forced into a coffin with a tube sock shoved in my mouth and I wasn't having it. I begged her to let me out. I was hyperventilating, sobbing, and squirming all around while still pinned down by the boobs. It was terrifying. But, instead of being sweet like she had been before, the MRI lady started yelling at me. She told me that I was her last patient of the day, that she wanted to go home, and that if I didn't get this done today, I would not be able to start chemo on Monday. I am not one to beg, but oh my gosh, did I ever. I begged her to let me out to readjust and regroup, all while apologizing profusely. I was in a full-blown panic. This experience became the bright and shining example of what the rest of my treatment would look like. Moving forward I knew I would constantly have to do things that terrified me, if I wanted to live.

As a result of my freak-out, the cranky MRI lady begrudgingly brought me out of the tube, removed the boob clamps (finally!), and let me up. I just needed a few moments to crack my back, pull my hair back, and catch my breath. We used Coban elastic bandage wrap as both a ponytail holder and a headband. To feel less constricted, I took off the oversized hospital socks and opened up the hospital gown down the back. Within a few minutes, I was back on that sliding table, face down, with the MRI lady re-locking my boobs back into place. The amount of mental fortitude it took to lie there and remain still took at least 780% of my willpower. And the amount of nonsense going through my head during that 40-minute MRI was obscene. I thought about how much it would suck to die young, how much I would miss my kids, and how badly I did not want to quickly, and permanently, be confined inside a coffin. I wished I had the superhuman ability to simply stand up with a roar and make that machine crumble around me.

I'm pretty sure that I counted every single second of that scan. It took about 20 minutes to do the first part of the imaging, before I was injected with the dye. Once administered I could feel the cold liquid coursing through the veins in my right arm. And then things got worse. The dye completely turned my stomach, which meant I was lying face down, with my nose about a millimeter away from the table below me, thinking I was going to throw up. A lot. But because I was desperate not to repeat the experience, I told myself that even if I threw up and my nose and chin were resting in my own vomit, I would not move. I had to get through it so I wouldn't have to do it again. It was a living nightmare.

Fortunately, after a few minutes, the nausea subsided, and I was able to remain still until the MRI was over. When she told me I was done, I lost it again. I could not stop sobbing and hyperventilating. It was the culmination of the worst week of my life and, hopefully, will hold the title as the worst hour of my entire life. For a Type-A person like me, that big of a breakdown was a big deal. When I was done, I had no interest in going back to the little changing room to put on my regular clothes. I literally wanted to sprint out of the building in that goofy gown to get away from the MRI. Remember that scene in the movie *Pee Wee's Big Adventure* when he runs out of the burning pet store, holding a bunch of snakes that he rescued in each hand, screaming? That's what I felt like doing. To me, the face down MRI experience was akin to being buried alive and I was desperate to escape that machine. That room. That entire building. But of course, instead of running and screaming, little Miss Type-A went back to the changing room, put on her clothes, and walked out like a mature adult. It definitely wasn't what I wanted to do, though.

I think it's important to know that all cancer cases are different. In fact, I have learned that each is as unique as a snowflake or fingerprint. Even within the exclusive realm of breast cancer, there are many different triggers, varieties, genetic factors, tumor sizes, and locations within the breasts. Some patients have it spread to their lymph nodes while others have it spread to their organs.

Some are metastatic and some are not. Some have successful treatment options and some do not. Please keep that in mind as you continue reading my story. I am only referencing my personal experiences, my treatments, and my outcomes.

March 8. Friday.

This was another fun morning. I woke up around 6 a.m. to head to Lake City Medical Center, about 40 miles north of Gainesville, to have my port-a-cath or "port" put in. If you're unfamiliar with a port, it's a small bottle-top shaped device attached to a catheter that is guided into a large vein above the right side of the heart. This is known as the superior vena cava. The top of the bottle-shaped device is made of a thin silicone that needles can penetrate without tearing. Instead of constantly sticking arm veins, ports become a cancer patient's go-to location for blood draws and fluid infusions. Mine was surgically installed underneath my collar bone, between my midline and my right shoulder. While having my port inserted seemed like a simple process, this was real surgery, under real anesthesia, with my very real surgeon, Dr. Sarantos. I normally would have chosen to have surgery at one of the local hospitals, but Dr. Sarantos was working in Lake City that week and I was willing to go anywhere to get this cancer-killing show on the road.

When I checked in and was brought to my pre-op bed, I cried. When I put on my blue gown and gigantic hospital socks, I cried. When they started the IV, I cried. Finding a trend here? Yep. I was a weepy mess. Cancer is extraordinarily stressful and makes even the most mundane medical procedures feel uber intense. Besides being stressed, I also had the good fortune of being hungry because I wasn't allowed to eat after midnight the day before. Since normally I'm someone who eats pretty small amounts at a time, hunger turns into "hanger" fairly quickly, and often, for me. I couldn't wait to be sedated so I wouldn't have to feel hungry anymore. Another odd thing I experienced prior to the procedure was the big concern for me "falling." Two weeks prior, I was running races and considered a very athletic girl. But on this day, they had given me a bright yellow wrist band with the word "fall risk" on it. What? Really?

I'm a fall risk? And there was also a big sign next to my pre-op bed that said, "Don't fall, Call!" Twilight Zone.

Before surgery, the anesthesiologist came in to give me the low down on my sedation. Sounded great. I asked him to sedate me quickly so I could stop feeling hangry, but no dice. Dr. Sarantos also came in for a pre-operation chat. He began by giving me the results of my MRI. Thankfully it only confirmed the scary things we already knew about, and there was no sign of cancer anywhere else. There was, however, a little something strange on my right breast. But the radiologist deemed it not to be concerning. I could have chosen to freak out over that news, but I decided to just trust my doctors instead. He reminded me how the port procedure would go and then left to prepare for it. His bedside manner was very reassuring and I knew he was going to take excellent care of me. He's considered the most competent guy with a knife in town. Before I was wheeled into the O.R., I asked Rob to greet me with a Diet Coke and French fries when I woke up. Yes, I know. Not a healthy choice. Whatever. That's what I wanted.

Things progressed quickly after that. I was pushed in my bed to the operating room, where I remember moving on to a different table. And that's about all I remember. Lights out for Fitz Koehler; I went straight to la-la land. That's the beauty of surgery under sedation. You don't have to actually experience any of it. It's weird to think about lying there, completely unconscious, while a room full of (mostly) strangers maneuvered my scantily clad body around to cut it open and insert an odd little device. What made it all better, though, was that at the helm was a brilliant surgeon who I truly believed cared about me and my health.

I think it's rude that they try to wake up sedated patients so quickly. I knew there was some sort of rhyme or reason to it, but it was the best sleep ever and I resented that quality sleep being disrupted. My memory is a bit foggy, but after the surgery, a nurse from the O.R. woke me up. For some reason I fixated on his beard and apparently told him how much I liked it about 7,342 times before I passed out again. That probably got old for him real fast. But thank goodness I liked his beard instead of disliking it, because it would have been a really rough morning for that guy if I kept negatively harping on his face. When I rewoke up in the recovery room and saw Rob, the first words out of my mouth were, "Pew! Pew!" I have no idea where that came from, but it became the official sound of cancer-killing from there on out. #PewPew would stick with me throughout my treatment. More importantly, when I went back to the recovery room, Rob greeted me with my Diet Coke, some French fries, and a bonus chocolate chip cookie. I only ate a few bites, but they were very satisfying. Besides the fresh, but razor-thin incision on my upper chest area, my port gave the appearance that I had a bottle top or big button under my skin. I was told that ports are usually pretty hard to see on larger patients, but since I was so lean, mine would be fairly pronounced. It was. I didn't really care about its appearance, though. I did, however, not enjoy feeling the weird little catheter under my skin. That creeped me out. We checked out and headed for home around noon.

A few hours later, I was at another facility for an echocardiogram. One of the things they would keep a close eye on throughout chemo was my heart. Heart damage is a realistic consequence of many chemotherapy drugs, so this first echo grabbed my baseline of heart function. I'd go in to get one every three months to monitor any changes. I'm a huge fan of my heart and this process is completely non-invasive and non-scary, so I was always happy to go have it done.

March 9. Saturday.

This weekend was reserved for quality time with family and we were joined by my very-concerned mother-in-law and niece, Abby. Our plan was to go out to lunch and then check out some wigs. But before we left the house, I uploaded my video entitled "I have breast cancer" to my Fitzness Facebook page and hit "publish." I figured it was time since things were about to get rolling. After publishing the video I turned my phone on silent so that I wouldn't be distracted. Lunch was filled with big laughs and clever conversations, and then we were off to Archer Beauty. My heart wasn't really into wig shopping, but I wanted to take the edge off by creating some fun experiences with my kids. I thought it might be fun or funny. Instead, it was just hard.

For starters, wig shopping around here isn't very impressive. I'm not sure exactly where great wig shopping exists, but Gainesville, Florida, definitely isn't the place. Especially for a young-ish white girl. Here's why: there are two choices of shops. One shop is Especially for Women, which carries all sorts of things for women who are nursing, enduring cancer treatments, dealing with alopecia, etc. It's wonderful, but the wigs in this place seem to cater to the 60+ crowd. Lots of short and sassy cuts. They had catalogs with longer, more youthful options, but not much in the store to try on. The other choice is called Archer Beauty. Archer Beauty caters to people of color. I've shopped there frequently for lashes, barrettes, and hair bands, and it's been perfect for those things. Unfortunately, when it comes to wigs, almost all of their options are for black chicks. What Archer Beauty didn't have, was a ton of options for me. I was hoping for something longish and blonde, similar to the hair that was soon to fall out, leaving my head lonely. It would have been great if they had something that would allow me to look, and feel, like myself.

When we arrived at Archer Beauty and headed toward the wig section, Lynn, the wig lady greeted me warmly. I told her what was going on and what I was hoping to find. She was incredibly kind and, when she sat me in a chair in front of a mirror, she asked if she could pray on my head. Of course, she could. I'm not a big church girl, but who in their right mind would reject prayers and warm wishes? Not me! I've received plenty through this journey, and I have been grateful for every single one. When she was done praying, she explained quite honestly that she really didn't have too many options for me, but she went in her back room to bring out what she had. I only learned a few things about wigs, but most memorable in my mind is that

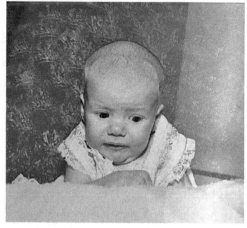

I had been bald once before. It doesn't look like I enjoyed it.

I could choose between fake hair and real hair. Real hair is more expensive and is supposed to be super easy to wash and style, and it lasts a long time. But I have to be honest. The thought of having someone else's hair draped across my shoulders creeped me out. I have a few girlfriends with wigs made from real hair, and they love them, but I was not interested.

After I bought the required wig cap, Lynn brought out several blonde wigs for me to try. A wig cap is kind of like pantyhose for your head and you put it on before you affix your wig. A few of the wigs were straight and blonde like I wanted, but the color was definitely not my blonde and not the type of blonde that made me feel pretty. One was short and curly like Shirly Temple. It was preposterous, but I tried it on so everyone could have a big laugh. Once they calmed down, I yanked it the hell off. I was trying so hard to be upbeat and smiley for my kids, but with every wig I tried on I felt sadder and sadder. Each one broke my heart a little more and left me crying pathetically in my weird little wig chair. Nothing allowed me to look like me and, on top of that, they were all really uncomfortable. I couldn't imagine walking out into the world wearing any of them. Finally, I agreed to try on a long reddish/brownish fake hair wig. Ginger and Parker were very excited about it because it reminded them of superhero hair. I think it was a bit like the X-Men's Jean Grey (The Phoenix). I had zero interest in ever wearing it, but at $40, it was super cheap and I bought it in an effort to cap the experience on a positive note. I walked out of that store knowing that I would never wear that wig, or any other for that matter. Wigs felt weird, they made me sad, and I knew that absolutely zero people on planet earth would ever believe they were my real hair. Bald would be my fate, and I embraced it. Plus, men didn't hide their bald heads. Why would I? I wouldn't!

Walking past the hair bands in that store ripped my heart out. I never thought the site of a ponytail holder would be so painful, but it was. They still send a dagger through my chest. I loved my swinging ponytails so much and I miss them desperately. Ugh. This was harsh.

When I returned home, I decided to check out the responses to my video upload on Facebook. The feedback was staggering. I'm pretty sure within just a few hours there were at least 500 or so sweet and supportive messages from friends around the world. Those messages continued to come and still do. The outpouring of love was humbling and certainly made me feel like I must have done something right along the way to gather so many wonderful people into my world.

As I mentioned, I didn't want unsolicited advice. While well-intentioned, I didn't like anyone who wasn't my doctor sending me pointers on this or that. I didn't want to hear the random thoughts or experiences of thousands of people. Much of it was unnecessary and downright depressing. I had a world-class medical team, and I was going to rely on them for guidance. However, I did choose a few particular friends, including Cheryl Tyrone, to rub antennas with. A couple of months before I found my lump, my friend Helen Legall, a retired police officer who used to work with Rob, was diagnosed. I remember my heart dropping out when I heard she had breast cancer. Helen is such a sweet woman and the news really bothered me. Never in a million years did I think I would end up in the same boat. Like Cheryl, Helen served as a guide, sounding board, and source of comfort. She had a different type of breast cancer and was receiving different chemo drugs, but she had gone first and had plenty of experience to share. She was always there for me and I tried to do the same for her. Both she and Cheryl constantly checked in on me, sent cards, and were all together exactly what I needed.

March 10. Sunday.

We went to see the movie *Captain Marvel* as a family. It was a sweet, low-key day together and I was grateful for it. Something I'd like to address here is that at the time of my diagnosis I became really uncomfortable with pink ribbons, which are the symbolic emblem for breast cancer and finding its cure. I'd worn these ribbons many times before in support of the cause and other women I care about. But suddenly I wanted nothing to do with them. That, of course, made me feel like a bad person. Tons of people had rallied behind those ribbons for fundraising and awareness and cures. Why wouldn't I just glom on? I didn't know, but the second I was diagnosed, I steered clear. I would eventually figure my feelings out, but at this point, I just did what felt right for me. So many people would eventually give me gifts with pink ribbons on them: shirts, pins, scarves, and bags. All very sweet and lovely. Ginger enjoyed all of it.

March 11. Monday.

I woke up eager to start the cancer killing process, but was understandably nervous about my first day of chemo. I had asked a few of my friends about their experiences and their responses didn't make things sound too bad. Both Cheryl and Helen had been treated with a chemotherapy drug nicknamed "The Red Devil." I'd heard about that one before and feared it, but neither of my sweet friends had too hard of a time with it. They both described feeling tired and mousy for a few days post-chemo, but those were consequences I could deal with. Since, in my mind, the Red Devil was worse than what I was going to get - I figured I should be fine too. Boy was I wrong. But it was probably better that I was a bit ignorant going in.

Since I was going to be the first to arrive and the last to leave daily, I was told to bring a bunch of stuff to chemo with me to keep me comfortable and entertained. I remember packing my iPad to watch Netflix, a snarky coloring book from a friend, MadLibs from my daughter, snacks, a pillow, blankets, and my laptop in case I wanted to get some work done. Chemo days would start with an appointment with Dr. Gordan or his nurse practitioners. We would talk about my health, they'd do a quick check-up, answer questions, and then release me to walk across the building for chemo. Once there, my port would be accessed, blood would be drawn, and if my blood counts looked good, the doctor would give permission for the pharmacists to whip up my drugs for infusion. Good times.

Still secretly convinced that I was going to drop dead soon, I again asked Dr. Gordon whether or not he thought I would beat this. At that point, he threw out some powerful statistics. He said that 93% of all breast cancer cases are curable and that mine was specifically curable because I caught it early, and HER2 positive and estrogen-positive breast cancer is well-understood. He was calm, cool, and brilliant, so I decided to stop thinking I was going to keel over quickly. With his permission, Rob and I headed over to the infusion room where I met my chemo nurse, Lisa "Lilly" Stoll. When I arrived at chemo, I checked in with the head nurse, who distributed patients like a hostess at a restaurant. Thank goodness I was distributed to Lilly. She was everything I needed her to be. She greeted me with a "Hey baby. Welcome to the Lilly pad. Go ahead and build your nest." She was kind and warm and asked me to choose my chair. The huge infusion room had about 60 recliners, but they were divided into small sections that each nurse was responsible for. I chose one way in the back of the room because I wanted to be as isolated as possible. I was accustomed to people seeing me as strong and vibrant, and I didn't want to give that up. Cancer was making me a bit of a hermit.

Unfortunately, alone is not what I ended up with. As Rob and I walked to my chair, he ran into a fellow police officer whose wife was also being treated for breast cancer. They greeted each other and introduced us. I'll call his wife, "Sally." Sally was very nice, and I genuinely felt for her, but this wasn't a great day for us. As soon as we said hello, Sally decided to dump all of her breast cancer horror stories on me. She told me about how hard the treatments had been, how her cancer had gone away and then returned, where it had spread, etc. The more she talked, the higher my anxiety levels rose. I just couldn't fathom how anyone would think that sharing this type of information with a brand-new cancer patient would be a good idea. Again, I felt for Sally and rooted for her, but this wasn't awesome. My situation was already scary and stressful, and she was making it worse. It would have been better if she had wished me luck and saved the bitch session for another day. Thankfully, Lilly saw what was going on, pulled me out of the conversation, and put me in my chair. She also rotated my chair a little bit away from the others, so I could have some breathing room. Lilly was my hero. As the months went on, she would continue to rescue me in different ways.

Rob joined me and was also surprised and disappointed by the conversation we'd just had. But we moved on quickly. I remember him asking me if I was ready. That's like asking someone if they are ready to step in front of a train or leap off a cliff. Sure, I was eager to start annihilating cancer, but I wasn't necessarily ready for the poisoning to begin and for life as I knew it to end. For sickness, fatigue, baldness and Lord knows what else. Still, I nodded my head and we got the scary show on the road. The first thing Lilly had to do was access my port. That means she had to poke the needle through my chest and into the port, which led to the catheter that pushed the drugs directly toward my heart. Once she got that needle into me (which would stay there for the day like an IV would in your arm), she could then administer the drugs, draw blood, etc. For the record, having a needle poked into the soft spot in your upper chest does not feel very good. Not good at all. It would have been far less painful to have the needles go into my arm, but that wasn't really an option. Lilly made the best of it though. She preempted each poke by spraying my port with icy cold freezy stuff that was supposed to numb the area. In my opinion, it doesn't numb anything, but it did serve as a mild distraction, so I always agreed to it. Then she told me to "cough on three" and she'd stick the needle through my chest on "three." She counted, "One, two, three," and instead of coughing, I squealed, "Fuck!" I wasn't good at following directions. The new game plan became Lilly counts to three and I'd curse loudly while she stabbed me in the chest. I would continue to curse my face off through almost every aspect of my treatment. Oh, and as you could probably guess, I cried.

Once my port was accessed, things got moving. Lilly drew blood and then sent it to the lab in the next room. Within 10 minutes, the results of my blood work came back and Dr. Gordan approved me for chemo. Next up, I was given a bag of anti-nausea meds, some Benadryl, and some steroids. I was also told to take a special anti-nausea drug called, "Varubi." Varubi is apparently a must-have medicine that helps with my type of treatment. Varubi also became a total pain in my rear. At $500 a pill, or something like that, my two Varubi pills were to be delivered the day before each round of chemo via a popular express shipping company. The main problem with Varubi had nothing to do with Varubi itself. The problem was that the shipping company screwed up its delivery five out of six rounds. That morning, poor Rob had to drive 60 miles south of our house to fight for my Varubi pills, which were trapped in a dis-

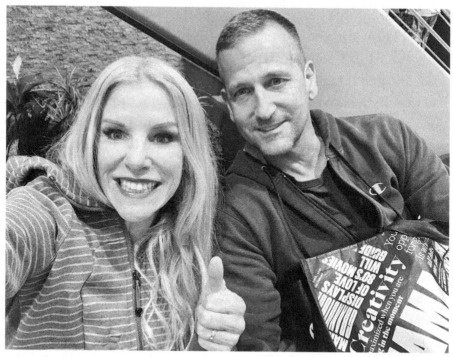

Rob and I waiting for my first round of chemo.

tribution center. This was not the way we wanted to start out my chemo regimen. It was a huge aggravation that continued on for months. I was continuously frustrated and it made me sad for the frail elderly patients who couldn't battle it out like we regularly had to.

Nevertheless, once the pre-meds were delivered, I would start my actual chemotherapy. I received each drug individually over a predetermined amount of time and, sometimes, I would have to just hang out and be observed. The drugs were given individually so in the event that I had an allergic reaction, they would know precisely what caused it. Apparently, the drugs I received had a high likelihood of causing an allergic reaction, so many preventative measures were taken. I was warned upfront that I should notify Lilly immediately if I had any weird feelings. Itching, chills, hives, shakes, stabbing pains, numbness, etc., I'd need to say something. Another patient had an allergic reaction on my first day, and the response was impressive. The nurse quickly stopped the infusion and every single nurse in the room swarmed on that patient. Then one of the doctors hustled out. And then the paramedics arrived. Oy! It was a mega-big deal. The kind of big deal I wanted nothing to do with. And, to be honest, even though I would come to fear my chemo drugs, I still wanted them. An allergic reaction would have caused my doctor to put me on a lesser drug, and second-best was not an option for me. I wanted to obliterate every nasty cancer cell in my body. No mercy!

All of my IV bags hung on my very own IV pole alongside a piece of paper with my infusion schedule. The schedule detailed the order in which I was to receive each drug, and for how long Lilly would set the drip. Mine read like this:

- Varubi - orally
- Benadryl - 5 minutes
- Aloxi - anti-nausea - 5 minutes
- Decadron - steroid - 5 minutes
- Perjeta - 60 minutes
- Observation - 60 minutes
- Herceptin - 90 minutes
- Taxotere - 60 minutes
- Carboplatin - 30 minutes
- Benadryl - 20 minutes
- Neulasta!® Onpro®

It was weird sitting there with an IV pole. It was even weirder walking around with that IV pole on wheels. While I did lots of sitting, chemo made me do lots of walking … to the bathroom. My tiny little bladder could only take so much liquid at a time, and then I had to get up and go to the loo. It's funny. There's a little half-inch ledge going from the infusion room into the restroom. All of us patients had to fight to get our poles over that ledge. From the place I would eventually sit on a regular basis, this became my entertainment. My personal technique for conquering that ledge was a kick. Kind of like when you want to chip a soccer ball. I would just kick the wheels of my pole in an upward motion and my pole would jump into the bathroom. It worked for me. Everyone else seemed to have their own unique methods, and I enjoyed watching most of them win the battle.

My childhood friend, Nicole Zimmerman Bodlack, came to visit me, which was both comforting and fun. Nicole and I go way back to elementary school, and we love each other so much. I know it pained her and many of my other friends to see me go through this tough time. Jennifer Sen also came by with love and support. I met Jen and her husband, Arup, when their son AJ was taking a hip hop dance class with Parker when the boys were just three years old. They've since become our chosen family and they've supported us nonstop through this year of crisis. While Lilly originally told me that I couldn't have guests during chemo, she always let me have them. She could tell I was stressed, and it was a simple way to keep me happy. Rob brought us lunch, and then I quickly passed out for a few hours. Lilly gave me pillows and warm blankets, which came straight out of a blanket heating oven. This made me feel fancy, like Oprah Winfey. I remember Oprah saying long ago that her housekeepers warmed her blankets every night before she crawled into bed. So uptown! The Benadryl I received practically knocked me out, as I'm such a freaking lightweight, so I made good use of my semi-cozy setup.

One of the weirdest side effects arrived instantly. When I stood up at some point to go to the bathroom, I noticed my quadricep muscles were really sore. Sore as if I had recently done a bazillion lunges or climbed Mount Everest. I hadn't. My quads had no reason to be sore, but they were, and it was odd. Even odder was that the soreness didn't go away for five solid months. That's right. My quads remained permanently sore for the entire course of mean chemo. Do you have any idea how often you stand up or sit down in a day? Imagine if every single time you did that, your legs screamed, "STOP!" That was me, and I had no clue this soreness would be long-lasting.

My day started at 9 a.m.and ended around 6 p.m. when Lilly woke me up to give me my Neulasta Onpro and send me on my way. It was a long day and as I was warned, I was officially the last patient to leave the infusion room. Neulasta may sound familiar to you as it's heavily advertised on TV. I can tell you that it's painful but clever, weird, and funny. Its purpose is to boost white blood cells, which can really take a hit during chemo, and lower a patient's risk of infection. Ideally, this medicine is given about 24 hours after chemotherapy, but to help people avoid a second trip back to their doctor for it (some people travel many miles for treatment), they attach this device to the patient, and

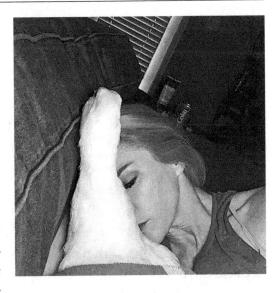

Passed out on the couch napping with Handy after chemo #1.

then it self-administers the shot at the appropriate time. Neat, right? I think so. When I was originally told about Neulasta, I was informed that the oval three-dimensional device would have to be attached to my stomach. That was not going to happen. I instantly refused because getting a shot in the tummy sounded horrible. But since I didn't have much belly fat, I was offered the opportunity to have it attached to the back of my arm instead. I was far more comfortable agreeing to that. After watching a little instructional video on an iPad, Lilly affixed it to my left arm with sticky tape, and then hit a "start" button. Then I was told to wait for the injection. The waiting period took about 90 seconds and was very strange. There was a ticking sound that preempted the eventual "Snap!" that I would hear and feel as the catheter was spontaneously injected into my arm. It was scary and somewhat painful, but also kind of comical.

Wobbly on my feet, Rob drove me home, where I was greeted with warm hugs by my sweet Ginger Bean and Parker Beans. I immediately curled up on the couch and was given my adorable duck, Handy, to nap with. Cuddling with Handy on the couch that evening post-chemo was

EXACTLY what the doctor ordered. She put her bill on my head before falling asleep while I slept. I felt pretty lucky to have her.

March 12. Tuesday.

The next two days were just as Cheryl and Helen had described. I felt a bit mousy and fatigued, but I was able to do basic things like running errands and meeting my friend Kim Cinque for lunch. I consider Kim the Patron Saint of Gainesville. She simply loves to dote on people and does so much work for those in need. We ate at one of our favorite places, McAllister's Deli, where I'd typically get an unsweet tea. But when my tea was delivered, it tasted pretty bad. I ended up telling the waiter that something was wrong with it and requested water instead. I'm an idiot, because there was absolutely nothing wrong with the tea. The problem was with me. My taste buds had apparently self-destructed, and nothing would taste right for a long, long time. I knew it would happen, I just hadn't realized it would happen this quickly. Bummer. From this point on, everything I ate tasted like it was covered in black dirt. Not brown or red dirt. Black. Why? Everything tasted bland with a weird texture, as I imagine black dirt would taste. I've been able to put very distinct imagery to a lot of my experiences. By the way. Black dirt tastes gross. Don't try it.

I also got to experience the beeping and administration of my first Neulasta shot. While chilling on the couch around 8:30 p.m., my arm started making sounds as though a little bomb was about to explode. The injection was made, the catheter automatically ejected from my arm, the red light came on, and Rob removed the device for me. Overall, not too bad of an experience.

March 13. Wednesday.

Waking up with a splotchy red rash on my face and neck didn't make me feel beautiful. It wasn't painful, but the red spots certainly weren't attractive and I did my best to cover them up with foundation. Also, for those who are interested, I deliberately didn't exercise during the days after chemo. I walked Piper a bit but didn't hit the gym as it made sense to give my body some time to rest. I was ignorantly hopeful that things were as bad as they would get, and it was about this time that I set some mini-goals for myself. Of course, being cured and never having breast cancer return was the most important thing on my list. But I felt like setting and achieving a few mini-goals might be fair as well. These goals were as follows:

- Avoid being hospitalized.
- Keep my muscles.
- Keep my lashes.

To me, these were very reasonable wishes, and I was really hoping to escape this experience having achieved them.

I'll reiterate that I was floored by the outpouring of love I received when I shared my bad news. But with the flood of goodwill, I also experienced some curious responses. Many very well-intentioned people reached out with a message that looked something like this: "Hi, Fitz. I hope you are well. Just wanted to let you know that my mom died of breast cancer. Sorry." Ummm. WHAT? Why would you tell me that? I mean, I know these individuals were making an effort to connect to my situation. But, really? I was trying very hard to get the lethality of my disease off of my mind. I didn't need a ton of little reminders that I might just die after all. Believe it or not, this happened with great frequency. Some would greet me with a big smile and say, "My aunt died of breast cancer last year!" Was I supposed to say, "Cool! Thank you?" Nah. I get it. Everyone knows someone who's died of cancer, and most people know someone who lost their life specifically to breast cancer. It's awful. What I'm hoping you'll take away from this rant is my plea for you NOT to do this to another patient. If they have a disease that you've heard terrible things about, keep the scary stuff to yourself. Instead, try to be positive. I managed these insensitive remarks fairly well because I'm sturdy. Other patients might have ended in despair as a result. Please keep that in mind.

March 14. Thursday.

I woke up feeling pretty weird. My stomach was kind of cranky, and I wasn't really sure what was going on. To add a little excitement to my mix, I was told to stop taking my birth control pill the day I started chemo. I had been on it for years to prevent painful ovarian cysts, but since my breast cancer was estrogen positive, I had to stop. Dr. Gordan told me that stopping the pill would cause me to get my period, but that it would likely be the last one I'd get during treatment. Fair enough. All day, as my tummy was feeling unsettled and irritable, I couldn't figure out if the cause was the chemo or my period. Either way, I was starting to feel lousy. Lousy enough that when I picked Parker and Ginger up from school and they asked what we were having for dinner, I died inside. I just thought, "I can't do dinner. I can't do food!" I remember starting to panic internally as I was feeling worse with every minute that went by. But as I was fretting about dinner on the way home, the most amazing thing happened. Out of the blue, my neighbor Becky texted to see if her husband Ron could bring us something from a local Mexican restaurant since he was headed that way. I promise you, I'm one of those people who has a hard time accepting help, but on this occasion, I quickly and gratefully accepted.

I remember sitting at the table with my family while they ate. Even though I couldn't touch a bite, I was so happy they had a nice meal. And then it happened. My stomach literally exploded. Think violent stomach bug meets tequila hangover. I was what they call "chemo sick", and it was horrendous. Over the years, we've all seen movies and TV shows where cancer patients are stuck in the bathroom, ill. That was me. Sadly, I would remain that sick person for the next five months. I had no idea that I was in for such a constant and lengthy battle. Ignorantly, I really thought the exploding would stop sooner rather than later. I thought it might just go away. It didn't.

In hindsight, this was probably the point in which I should have reached out to Dr. Gordan to let him know what was going on. After all, he'd given me his email address and his personal cell phone number. Instead, I just chose to suffer. Like an idiot. I remember thinking that I was on chemo, and I was supposed to be sick, so why would I bother him to tell him that? That weekend was a nightmare. Exploding led to dehydration, which led to extreme fatigue, lethargy, dizziness, and all sorts of nonsense. I almost fell a few times. Where was my "fall risk" wristband? Thankfully I never hit the ground. I had anti-nausea meds, but I refused to take the strongest ones because I didn't want to be knocked out. Unfortunately, the others weren't working.

On a goofy note, Rob and I kept thinking that getting me up to get moving would be a good idea. We kept trying to go for little walks thinking that activity and fresh air might help. I look back and laugh at our stupidity, but what did we know? At one point, I think I made it past three houses on a walk before tapping out. I simply needed to lie flat and stagnate. Moving was making me feel worse. On Monday morning, after a 3 a.m. explosion, I couldn't take it anymore and gave in to my sickness. Feeling pathetic, I emailed Dr. Gordan. I told him how sick I'd been since Thursday and asked if there was anything he could do to help. I woke up to his email asking me to come in as soon as possible to see him and get some IV fluids. I was so grateful that he had plans to help me feel better. I was desperate.

March 18. Monday.

As we spoke in the exam room, I told Dr. Gordan that I had to get on a plane Friday morning to announce the Los Angeles Marathon. Instead of telling me to stay home or cease traveling, he told me that he was going to do everything he could to make sure that I was good to go. In fact, I'm pretty sure his exact quote was, "We need to get you on your feet!" Dr. Gordan is a half-marathoner who understands what I do and the value and joy my profession brings me. He wanted to help me keep living while I was undergoing treatment, and that meant the world to me. The plan was for me to come in for IV fluids every day until I left. And he would add Sustol (another preemptive anti-nausea shot) to my next chemo session. He also suggested a few over-the-counter meds to help stop my tummy from waging WWIII. I left our meeting and went straight to the infusion room for IV fluids.

I was hoping and expecting to see Lilly again, but as I checked in the nurse manager told me that I would be seeing Ben (not his real name) instead. I made an extra "pretty please" for Lilly but was told that she was too busy and that Ben was the only nurse available. Rob and I looked at each other with concern, wondering who Ben was, but we walked back to his section and took a seat. A few minutes went by with no sight of Ben, and then he started toward me. He looked to say, "Fee! Fi! Fo! Fum! I smell the blood of a noisy one!" Ben was big, strong, and kind of intimidating. What he was really lacking though, was a smile and a pleasant demeanor. Ben was in a rush and didn't offer any words of comfort or encouragement. In fact, he was awfully cold. I felt really sick and super sad, and I got zero empathy from Ben. When he tried to access my port, I naturally leaned my chest away. I was sternly scolded for doing so, and man, he leaned in so hard with his big sausage fingers and stabbed that needle right through the sore soft spot in my chest. Ouch! I felt like I was Uma Thurman in the *Pulp Fiction* overdose scene. Not fun at all. I'll tell you what. Ben didn't screw up any of the technical details of my care, but I certainly didn't feel cared for.

Quality, caring medical providers are so valuable. They have the power to make a difficult situation better or worse. While I was receiving my fluids, Rob emailed Dr. Gordan and told him I was not enjoying Ben's care. He asked if I could be permanently assigned to Lilly and our wish was granted. Rob swiftly told the head nurse lady about our new rules. Hooray for me! I returned each day to the Lilly pad, and the fluids worked their magic. I didn't stop exploding completely, but the dehydration and dizziness subsided, and that made all of the difference. Another set of wins came when I found out that 1) I do not carry any sort of genetic predisposition for breast cancer and 2) that it would not be necessary for me to have a full mastectomy and hysterectomy. This allowed me to breathe a huge sigh of relief.

One of the most powerful tools in my bag of Fitzy tricks is perspective. Many years before this all went down, I had a life-changing experience that has come in handy every time something has gone even remotely south. I was in the "10

Items or Less" checkout lane at my grocery store feeling rather impatient as a 946-year-old woman was writing a check for her 53 items. Of course I would never say anything, but I was internally irritated. As I stood there stewing, I caught a glimpse of a shiny Snow White gown on a tiny little girl who had a very bald head. I was pretty sure she had cancer and was enduring chemo, and it pained me to imagine what she and her parents must have been going through. And there I was, fretting over a long line. I decided that I would never again waste any of my energy being negative about trivial things. Instead, I would be wildly grateful for all of the positive things in my life. I have been able to successfully adhere to that plan. In fact, I've told this story on my podcast, The Fitzness Show, for years. When a wrench was thrown into my plans, I'd just take a deep breath and use my mantra, "It's not cancer!" And then I'd get over whatever was bothering me. But now, it was cancer. And do you know what? That dang perspective stuck around. Sure, I had cancer. But I wasn't a child with cancer and it wasn't my child with cancer. And, thankfully, I didn't have one of the far more typically lethal cancers. I had so much to be grateful for. Folks, I have had many difficult moments, days, weeks, and months because of cancer. I promise you this. Not ONCE did I wonder, "Why me?" Not ONCE did I complain about my situation. Perspective simply wouldn't allow it.

March 21. Thursday.

The second I found my lump, I began stressing over losing my hair. It was inevitable, but losing my long, fabulous golden locks was going to be torturous. Pre-chemo, losing loads of strands during a regular hair brushing never phased me. But now, I was fixated on each hair that left my head and kept wondering whether the real hair loss was starting or not. And 11 days after my first chemo session, it began. While brushing my hair before bed, there was a sudden and significant difference in the amount of hair coming out. It was more than upsetting, but I thought I could outrun it for the weekend. I wanted to try and get through the LA Marathon without drama. My strategy was to just not brush my hair anymore. Instead, I was just going to finger brush it and pat it down to avoid frizziness. That would probably prevent the hair from coming out too quickly. Right? Only temporarily.

From the start, Dr. Gordan told me that my hair would likely start falling out on day 11. His accuracy was astounding. He was clearly a wizard.

March 22. Friday.

I woke up, got dressed, and headed to the Gainesville Regional Airport around 4:30 a.m., still really sick, but reasonably functional. Concerned, Rob looked at me before I headed through TSA and asked, "Are you sure you want to do this? How are you going to do this?" With a blank stare, I shrugged my shoulders and responded, "I just will." I was going to Los Angeles. I boarded my plane and took my seat, but unlike normal, I was now a little concerned about sick people sharing germs with me. I whipped out the fancy surgical mask my massage therapist gave me and proceeded to become that weirdo wearing a mask on a plane. I made a solid effort to wear it, but since I'm claustrophobic and deal with a few respiratory issues, I couldn't keep it on for more than a second or two. I ended up trashing it and never wore a mask again. Oh well, I tried. Traveling was exhausting, but I was fortunate that when my plane touched down at LAX (Los Angeles International Airport), I was able to go straight to my hotel and sleep.

I normally announce the majority of my events alone, but on occasion, I also pair up with other announcers for larger events. My favorite person to co-announce races with is an absolute legend on the microphone, Rudy Novotny. He's also the person who got me started announcing races. I was teaching clinics for runDisney, which he had announced for many years at the time we met, and he was always very complimentary of my talent as a presenter. Coincidentally, I thought he was the best race announcer on the planet and still do. He's incredibly smart and charismatic, and we formed an almost instant friendship, sharing tales from our very similar endeavors on microphones. In the spring of 2014, he needed a co-announcer for the Orange County Marathon (OC Marathon) and reached out to see if I'd be interested. I was honest with my response, "I've never done it before, but I'd love to give it a try!" Rudy was confident I'd be a natural, so he connected me with race director Gary Kutscher, who checked out my work history and gave me a call. After a very short conversation, Gary invited me to announce his event with Rudy, and my career took a magical turn. Rudy was right. Announcing fit me like a glove and, within a few hours of my first "GO" at the OC Marathon, Gary had asked if I would return the following year. Within a few months, I had booked another handful of announcing gigs. The rest is history. Rudy and I have a very similar style and absolutely adore working together. We both bring high energy, humor, and love to the microphone. We genuinely care about our athletes, our race organizations, and everyone else who contributes. Our chemistry is undeniable, so we're often hired together, and over time, we've earned the nickname, "Team Noisy." Our loyal friends and fans in the running community have become "The Noisy Nation." Rudy and I simply couldn't have planned it any better. Besides being a blast to work with, he's genuinely one of my best friends, and I appreciate the lengths he went through to support me during this arduous year.

Back to Los Angeles. I was only able to go straight to my hotel after landing in LA because Rudy worked both of our shifts at the expo just so I could rest. Some of our races require us to host the shopping and bib pick-up parts of a race weekend, and this was one of them. I was running on fumes after my long day of travel, so getting to face-plant onto my bed instead of going to work was a huge relief. Before that face-plant, though, I finger brushed my hair, and all seemed well on my head. Point awarded to … Fitz Koehler!

March 23. Saturday.

Our morning began bright and early with the LA Big 5K and the LA 1/2K kids races. Most marathon weekends have some shorter races attached the day before the longer events. The LA Big 5K is short in distance, but it's big in participants; we had about 5,000. The air was cool and crisp, the people were enthusiastic, and it was all I needed to do my job. I'll share that there are a few things about race announcing that aren't the same for everyone, but they're particular to me.

First, I find the work easy. Easy in the way that it comes naturally to me, and I have zero fear of getting up in front of massive crowds. Helping folks have fun and making them feel special is in my nature, so those are the things that I find easy. The thing that makes it hard is the way that I do it. Some announcers sit on a stage at a start line and read a script. That's a minimally demanding way to work, but good for them. Everyone has their own methods. I can't help but put enormous amounts of energy into announcing. I may read a few bullet points, but for the most part, I talk big, I'm mostly unscripted, and I engage with my runners and walkers nonstop. The athletes and I do the start line experience together, and I believe that the more energy I give, the more likely they are to perform their best and have more fun. The finish line is similar. Many announcers sit on their perch and read names. Good for them. While I do a little of that too, I almost always spend a ton of time personally greeting runners in the finish line chute. I love to get them hyped up, to give them hugs, and oftentimes to run them through their finish lines. If you heard me welcome our final finishers of the day without actually seeing what was going on, you would likely think that I was welcoming in our winners. I want every participant to feel like a champion, so I give my everything from the time I'm handed a microphone until the last athlete is done. Again, it's effortless and fun for me, but it requires an enormous amount of energy. Some speakers are 30 watts. I'm a 300-watt speaker. Pre-cancer healthy Fitz always gave 110% to her races, and even she would normally need a few days to recover from that amount of output.

I tell you this because my game plan was to execute my race announcing efforts without sacrificing performance over the next year of treatment. The LA Big 5K was a fantastic start. To be specific, stepping onto my announcer stage was akin to plugging me in and flicking my "ON" switch. The feelings of fatigue and nausea I was experiencing just faded away as I turned my attention to our athletes. They pumped me full of adrenaline and that's exactly what I needed to bring: *the happy*. Team Noisy events are always a blast, but this morning was special. Our athletes were incredibly responsive to our shenanigans and once we yelled "GO," they ran by us with the biggest smiles, waving at us, shouting our names, and telling us they loved us. They were just oozing with joy and enthusiasm. I seriously never wanted the start of that race to end. What a gift for me to have this level of excitement in my life while I was enduring the calamity of cancer. Two days prior I was hooked up to an IV pole to help me cope with illness. And just as suddenly I was experiencing pure bliss. It took a good 10 minutes for all of the runners to cross the start line, and I felt so grateful to be there and be a part of such exuberance.

Rudy and I headed over to the nearby finish line, where the liveliness continued. I tell you, there is NOTHING dull about a race when we are working together. The gifts we bring to an event are returned to us a million times over. When we help our participants release their happy side and enthusiasm, we are the ones who get to consume it. It's endless fun and I never take one second or one runner for granted. Of the thousands of racers doing the LA Big 5K, the one who made me laugh the most, was the guy in the bright red inflatable T-Rex costume who was deflating as he crossed the finish line. We cried with laughter. As the final 5K athletes trickled in, I broke away from Rudy to go announce the kids' races. While I can gush about all of my athletes for a million reasons, the kids are the unmistakable stars. I believe the oldest in this event was about eight years old, and the youngest was about 14 months old. At the start line, the kids and I joke, pose for fun pictures, and do a heck of a lot of dancing. In fact, everyone gets forced to dance when I'm around. Kids particularly like it when I launch the Daddy Dance Party or get the mommies to shake their booties. At some point, I spontaneously and publicly told everyone to watch as our Conqur Endurance Group CEO Tracy Russell and COO Murphy Reinschreiber showed off their funky dance moves. Poor Tracy and Murphy were innocently standing on the sidelines to watch the kids run when I made the declaration. Thankfully, instead of firing me on the spot, they shook their thangs, and everyone loved it.

Saturday morning was a massive success, and I breathed a big sigh of relief that I was able to get through my first race post-chemo with flying colors. I also had enough energy to go announce the expo for a few hours and give Rudy a break. My stomach was still a mess, but I was able to manage it. Being at the expo allowed me to visit with hordes of my favorite runner friends and race directors. Since this was the first time anyone had seen me since my diagnosis, they were all extra sweet, concerned, and encouraging. When I got back to my hotel room that night, though, things with my hair started going downhill. An unusual number of strands were falling out, and I made the mistake of brushing it. This made enormous chunks come out. Panic was setting in. My hair was going to go, and soon. I went to sleep sobbing and hoping it would still be there in the morning.

March 24. Sunday.

This was one of the most emotionally taxing days of my life. My alarm went off at 4:30 a.m., so I could get ready and head directly to the marathon finish line. Since this race is a point-to-point course that takes our runners from Dodger Stadium to the Sea in Santa Monica, Rudy and I are separated at the beginning of the day. He works the start line alone and I wait for our initial athletes at the finish line. That's because some athletes can complete the course before a car can get from start to finish. Our first finishers, by the way, are our speedster wheelchair athletes. The hand cyclists can crush 26.2 miles in a little over an hour, so we divide and conquer to ensure everyone gets a warm welcome. Putting on make-up and fixing my hair in the morning was harrowing. Hundreds of hairs were falling to the bathroom floor and I was falling apart. My insides were twisting while my heart was breaking. I was trying desperately to control my emotions because I didn't want to have an ugly puffy face all day on my stage. But those efforts verged on futility. I was alone and I was melting down, all while telling myself I had to be a big girl and get myself to work. On a whim, I decided to document this experience on video, describing what it was like to have my hair fall out. Remember: I don't like sadness. But for some reason, I chose to put some key moments on camera in case I wanted to share them down the road. The video I captured as I choked back the tears is still gut-wrenching to watch. You can find it on my social media channels.

I arrived at the finish line with a fake smile on my face, greeting fellow staff members and volunteers cheerfully. I'm sure they would have allowed me to cry on their shoulders had they known what was going on, but that wouldn't have accomplished anything, and I had a job to do. A really fabulous job. When I got to my stage, I was desperately hoping for a great day, but instead got hit with the news that our sound team didn't show up on time and we didn't have any sound. Seriously. Nothing. Our chair athletes who deserved tons of celebratory love were going to be greeted with silence. I couldn't yell or get nasty with the sound team because that would have been completely unprofessional, and it wouldn't have fixed the sound situation anyway. Instead, I just sat there like a lady, alone in my announcing tower, grinding my teeth as our incredible chair athletes finished without any fanfare.

When Rudy arrived, I calmly, yet intensely, told him what had been going on. He meant well, but he almost lost his life when he told me to calm down. Cue head explosion. The man was lucky that I was so restrained, because I was being insanely restrained and profoundly calm given the circumstances. If I wasn't so disciplined, telling me to calm down would have triggered a nuclear bomb. But I was happy he was there and got past his dumb remark quickly. Eventually, we got some sound, but there was no bass. And that was annoying. Eventually we got about 87% of the sound we needed, and that was going to have to be good enough. Now, let this not reflect poorly on this incredible race. Stuff happens. Even to the best. This failure just happened to add to my already difficult morning. It was probably the only imperfection I've ever seen during the Los Angeles Marathon.

As the day went on, we had a really fun time welcoming in our athletes. We also had a really hard time because our windy beachfront stage, located about 10 feet up in the air, was soon covered with long blonde hair. It was coming out nonstop, and when I wasn't being cheery on the microphone, I was sobbing on Rudy's shoulder. It was devastating. Poor Rudy was working overtime to try and support me. When I was focused on our finish line, he was frantically sweeping piles of my hair off the stage so I wouldn't see them. He was also trying to deflect my attention by dancing silly and telling lots of jokes. It was the most schizophrenic day ever. I was genuinely joyful when distracted by runners and genuinely heartbroken when I was off of the mic for even a few minutes. Fortunately, my sunglasses ensured nobody saw my tears or had any clue I was struggling.

Throughout the day, dozens of my personal friends stopped by for hugs and sweetness before they crossed the finish line. Phil Cordeiro wore his Fitzness shirt and brought me a beautiful breast cancer pin. Connie Kosberg brought me a bouquet of flowers that she'd purchased

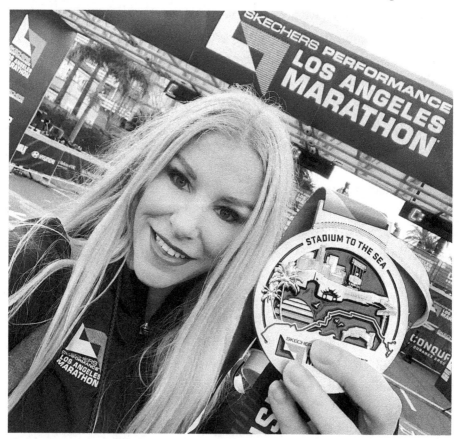

Every Los Angeles Marathon finisher went home with a medal and a hair.

from a street vendor at mile 20. So many others just brought lots of love. How lucky am I? In the midst of significant emotional trauma, I was being equally blessed with overwhelming joy.

At some point, my hair loss got so frustrating that I wanted to call a local stylist to just come and shave my head right there on the stage. It would have been wacky, but I was desperate to get it over with. The only thing that stopped me was the promise I made to Ginger that I wouldn't cut it without her. Losing my hair was a real sore spot for her, because she really liked having our long blonde hair in common. Unlike most teenage daughters who'd try to distance themselves from their mom, she was proud to be connected and that melted my heart. So I suffered through the experience and planned to deal with it when I returned home. At 3 p.m., our sound system was cut off and we were cut loose. I was certain that all 25,000 of our athletes went home with a beautiful medal and a single strand of Fitz hair. Talk about a weird souvenir! Then Rudy and I walked over to California Pizza Kitchen to grab a bite and rest our tired bodies. Poor man. I was sure that everyone in the restaurant thought he was being mean to me because I bawled in my booth through the entire meal. That night, I twisted my hair into a bun and cried myself to sleep.

March 25. Monday.

I woke up to the sobering reality that this would be the day that I would shave my head. It was hard to fathom as I had spent my entire life with long hair, but it was a task I could no longer put off. As I arrived at LAX, I texted my hairstylist to see if she would come to my house to take care of business that evening. She instantly agreed. I didn't want to bring my sadness into her salon, and doing it at home would provide the privacy I needed and the dignity I didn't want to give up. Kristen had become one of my best friends since she started doing my hair and I started training her in 2003. She is the classic southern woman: sweet like tea, strong, and capable.

My flight home provided further confirmation that I no longer had a choice. When I rose out of my plane seat to use the restroom, the amount of hair left behind was appalling. There were hundreds of long blonde strands on my seat and on the floor in the aisle. This would be upsetting with short hair, but mine measured 24 inches long! The mess was atrocious. I apologized to the woman sitting next to me and briefly explained my situation. She was sympathetic and assured me that she wasn't bothered, but I bet she didn't think it was fun to sit beside the super-shedder.

When I returned home from the airport with Rob, my kids and pets were waiting for me with lots of cuddles and love. Ginger was crying, and Parker offered sweet strength for support. While I knew that crying was reasonable in this situation, I was trying desperately to avoid completely breaking down. I remember how scary seeing my mom cry after her back surgeries was when I was a kid. Keeping my composure was impossible, but I did my best to hold it together.

It's amazing how many people have said, "It's just hair." And while that's true and I've always said that it was a fair exchange for my life, I'd like to tell those people SCREW YOU! We all like our hair, and almost nobody wants to go bald this way. Yes, it will most likely grow back, but the whole process is excruciating. If you ever think of telling a cancer patient or even someone with alopecia, "it's just hair" again please go whack your shin on a coffee table instead. It falls into the category of your dog dying and someone saying, "It's just an animal." Screw you! Rant over.

Kristen showed up around 8 p.m. and it felt like the Grim Reaper was walking through my door. To make things worse, it was the Grim Reaper that I had invited in! It was tormenting. After driving an hour to my house and seeing me cry, she offered to leave if I was having a change of heart. It was a very generous offer, but I knew it had to be done. The process of losing my hair naturally was too stressful and too messy. I had to rip off the bandage. And while many people suggested donating my hair, I had something more personal to do with it. Since he was an infant, Parker had always twisted the ends of my hair for comfort, and he asked if he could have it. Of course he could! It was a perfect choice, and it made me happy that he cared enough to want that part of me.

As we sat around our kitchen table, Kristen divided my hair into two parts, tied them into braids, and cut them off. I sat in the chair with my hands over my eyes weeping. Not as brave as everyone thinks I am. Then she asked me how I wanted to shave it. Ummm. Did I have a choice? Apparently, there are different lengths one can choose from with clippers. I didn't know. I had never shaved my head before. With Kristen's guidance, we decided to shave my head with a #2 guard, or ¼ inch, all around. Feeling the clippers slide over my scalp was a strange sensation. When Kristen was almost done, I heard the sweetest, "Mom, it looks kinda cool!," from

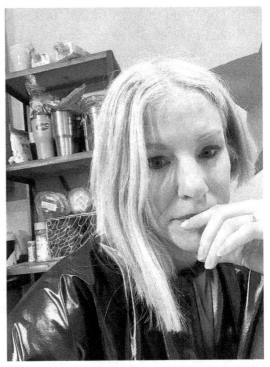

After my braids were chopped off.

Ginger. Parker agreed. There was a bunch of laughter and then I got the courage to go into our guest bathroom and look in the mirror.

Holy shit! Who in the world was that? I looked so different. Sure, my face was the same, but I had lost that soft halo surrounding it. It was shocking, to say the least. I certainly didn't love it, and I kind of didn't hate it. I just didn't recognize that girl anymore. I don't remember much more from that night other than more tears on my pillow as I fell asleep. To the outside world, I was making this all look easy and pretty much telling them that it was. The reality was that breast cancer and the treatments for it were wreaking havoc on me. How in the world did this happen?

March 26. Tuesday.

With my weird new hairdo, I woke up and headed straight in for IV fluids. My stomach was still a mess, and I was hoping they would help me recover before I headed back to California to announce the Encinitas

Half Marathon in a few days. Plus this was Parker's 14th birthday, and I wanted to celebrate it as a family. As soon as he came home, I forced a happy face, and we headed out for dinner, some bowling, and video games. My goal was to make sure that my cancer nonsense didn't infringe upon his special day. And I think we achieved that. Even though I was tired, and my tummy was a jerk, we were able to have some real laughs as he beat the pants off of us at air hockey. Mission accomplished.

March 29. Friday.

There I was, boarding another plane at 4:30 a.m. with a woozy look on my face. I wasn't feeling so hot, but nothing was going to keep me from my event. I'd had a few days to get used to my little buzz cut, but it was still very weird. I never felt embarrassed about it or had the impulse to hide it. I believe that embarrassment should only come when you do something wrong. Being treated with chemo didn't cause me any reason for shame. However, people looked at me in a new way. I didn't like people knowing or highly suspecting that I was sick. As a generic observation, I've noticed a ton of gorgeous black women who shave their heads for fashion and no one thinks anything of it. Many men also sport bald heads and we all just accept it as normal. But when a white girl does it, she often becomes the poster child for cancer. I don't think anyone thought I was just being edgy. Even though I still had a ¼ inch of hair, people started treating me differently. Nicely, but differently. When I landed in California, no one had seen my hair yet because I hadn't posted any pictures. I thought, if I'm going to debut a new hairdo, I might as well do it in front of 10,000 people, right?

March 31. Sunday.

At 50°F, the morning of the Encinitas Half Marathon and 5K was pretty cold for me.. Now, even with my long hair, I've always worn fuzzy hats to keep warm because they do a lot to help me maintain heat. But I made a decision that day. Though I didn't love the way I looked, I knew with 100% certainty that at least one or more of the runners in that crowd would one day face cancer, chemo, and hair loss. I decided that if I stood on a stage loud and proud with a shaved head, that maybe they too would have the courage to do so when the time came. Now, I completely support those who choose wigs, hats, and scarves. No judgment. But those things aren't for everyone. And they weren't for me that day.

Pre-race, we had a ton of friends stop by to share hugs, kindness, and support. Demarie Bottai and her Mermaid Squad of runners were wearing custom-made shirts that said, "Mermaids love Fitz." There was a "Mermen love Fitz" version as well. My high school friend and retired Marine Corps Lieutenant Colonel Brian Grana brought his hunky sons for hugs. Carrie DuShey brought me some beachy trucker hats. Our timers, Greg and Debbie Richards, brought me a ginormous gift bag, and Jeff and Tina Hauser brought me Diet Coke. The list goes on. Mostly, people let me know that they loved me and were rooting for me. It mattered so much. In fact, the outpouring of love had been nonstop since I revealed that I had breast cancer. Not everyone is as fortunate, and that fact was never lost on me.

My friend, Dana Sobotka, ran the 5K with her daughter, and after she crossed the finish line, I asked her to come to my stage for a visit. I met Dana the year prior when she ran the half marathon after completing her own breast cancer battle. Amongst the quick hugs and chit chat, she ended up sharing some mind-altering information. She asked how I was, and I responded, "Feeling decent enough, except my nose won't stop running." Now, this wasn't all that was going on, but I didn't want to go into the big stuff. I was pretty convinced that the constant dripping was some sort of allergic reaction like my rash, so I thought it would be a simple thing to mention. But Dana knew better. When I mentioned my runny nose, she said, "That's because your nostril hair fell out!" I was bowled over. Could that be true? Unfortunately, yes. She was spot on. My smooth and silky, hairless nostrils were the reason my nose was running. Not allergies. I simply had no hair in there to keep the sinus fluid in. What the hell? Nobody ever warned me of that! Sadly, my nose would continue to run for the rest of my treatment. And just so we're clear, this was not the standard type of running you experience when you have a cold. This was the splishy-splashy kind that dramatically falls like raindrops. Dare I look down at my shoes? Splish - splash. Look down to greet

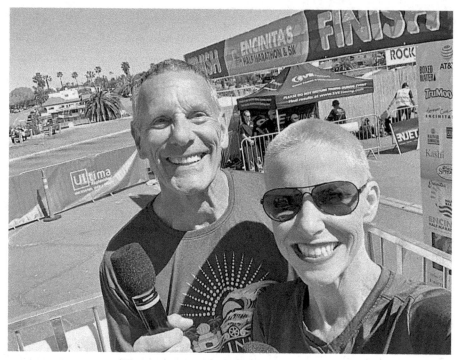

Rudy and I at the Encinitas Half Marathon finish line.

my dog? Splish - splash. It was ridiculous. I decided to stop taking allergy meds and stocked up on 57 million boxes of Puffs Plus tissues instead. I had no use for head wigs, but if I could've found teeny tiny nostril wigs to wear and stop my nose from running, I definitely would have worn them. Calling all inventors! Nostril wigs might be the new big thing.

Besides showing off my bald-ish head, I also debuted my hot red running tights. I figured if I didn't want people to look at my head, I could deflect their attention to my butt. I think it worked.

A few hours after the races were over, I boarded a red-eye flight home for chemo in the morning. Normally, I avoid red-eye flights at all costs because they simply ruin me. Trying to sleep in those awkward chairs is pretty close to impossible, but I boarded my first flight with strong ambitions to snooze the whole four hours from San Diego to Atlanta. Instead, I could only sleep for about 43 minutes, before pathetically squirming around in the dark until we landed. But it was the only way to keep me on schedule for chemo. As luck would have it, when I got home, I received an email that said I wouldn't be allowed to receive chemo this week because my liver numbers were too high. Ugh. That was annoying. While I wasn't looking forward to chemo, I definitely would not have taken the red-eye flight if I wasn't in any rush. But, something good came out of that flight. My mother had driven up to take care of me while my family was in New York for spring break. We were able to hang out, I got an extra week to recover, and I started to feel human again.

My mom was a great guest. She drove me around, came to some appointments with me, and forced me to take naps. We went out for meals, watched TV and played with Piper and Handy. She loved having a grand-duck. Even though she was taking care of me, I knew it meant a lot to her to get some quality time with her youngest child. And even though I am a full-grown, business-owning woman with a house, car, and kids, I will always be her baby. It has been painful for her to watch me go through this. She lives 300 miles away in Fort Lauderdale, so daily FaceTime reassurances that I was okay were a must. Sometimes my efforts failed, as these video calls would allow her to see that I looked horribly sick. Even when I would try to put on some makeup and freshen myself up, she could normally tell when I had bad days. Nonetheless, it was fabulous to have her visit, and I was okay having an extra week off before being poisoned again.

Fitzness Log

I exercised ferociously the nine days before my first chemo. I needed the mental escape, and I decided that the fitter I was before chemo started trying to knock me down, the better off I'd be in the long run. I wasn't wrong. Every ounce of the health and fitness we earn will benefit us in some way, shape, or form. My gameplan going into chemo #1 was to skip exercise for a few days and then maybe jump back into it a few days later. Ummm. Nope! My ignorance was adorable. By Friday, I was sick to my stomach and too weak to do anything energetic. The short little walks I tried to take did more harm than good, so I decided to choose rest and recovery over exercise. It wasn't what I wanted to do, but I had no choice. My healthy eating habits were also semi-thwarted. I wasn't chowing down on junk food, but my sensitive stomach wouldn't allow me to eat all of the fruits and vegetables I normally would. Plain potatoes, noodle soup and mac 'n' cheese were some of my go-to choices. Everything tasted horrible thanks to the black dirt phenomenon, but I leaned toward options without a lot of fiber, sugar, or spiciness to keep my tummy in check.

Chapter 4

I Can Do Hard Things

April 4. Thursday.

My itsy bitsy hair was still falling out and becoming very patchy, so I went into Kristen's salon for another shave. One would think it would have been easy since it was already buzzed so short, but it wasn't. Poor Kristen. I showed up asking for a cut and then cried all the way through it. This time, we decided to leave it as a #2 on top and shave it to a #1, or ⅛ inch, on the sides. It made me look like a male Air Force cadet and I really didn't like it. I ended up wearing a hat for the next few days until I could get back in with Kristen to fix it. I wasn't hiding bald. I was hiding a bad haircut.

April 5. Friday.

It had been almost four weeks since my first chemo and I felt pretty decent as I pulled into Savannah, Georgia to announce the Publix Savannah Women's Half Marathon and 5K. I arrived at my hotel and received a gift bag full of goodies from my race directors Rob Wells and Jonathon Sykes. They were concerned about me and I appreciated their thoughtfulness. Savannah is such a charming town, and my athletes are always full of sweet Southern energy. In many ways, the crowd is like others and in many others, it's not. I can say "y'all" and "bless your heart" on the microphone there and nobody looks confused. When I let anything like that slip out of my mouth on the west coast, I instantly feel like a doofus and the crowds look perplexed. I brought Rob with me for the weekend, so after stopping by the expo, we got to enjoy dinner with friends and took a trip to the Savannah Candy Kitchen, a famous sweet shop in the area.

April 6. Saturday.

I was pretty stoked to get to the start line in the morning. I love what I do, and it was nice to feel decent and get back to announcing. My friend Yesenia showed up wearing a custom Wonder Woman shirt with TEAM FITZ printed on the front. It was pretty unreal to have people do this for me. What I really loved though, was how normal my morning was. I was back to taking care of everyone else which is truly what makes me tick. My health was a non-issue, and I spent the morning running up and down the finish line chute supporting our runners and walkers. My friend Abdielia Sanz was back in Savannah for the second year, and it was especially great to see her. She's been undergoing cancer treatment for a while and makes bald look absolutely beautiful. I met her the year

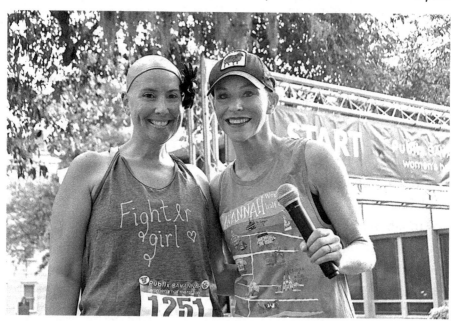

Abdielia Sanz makes bald look beautiful in Savannah.

prior as she finished our half. After making a royal stink over her finish, I spent some time getting to know her. She walks tons of half marathons each year and really serves as a role model for a lot of people, including myself.

April 8. Monday.

Since I was no longer questioning how horrible it was going to be, showing up for round #2 of chemo was pretty unnerving. On the one hand, I wanted the drugs because they would allow me to live. But on the other hand, I also feared them because I knew they were going to make me sick again. It was nerve-racking. In the days leading up to chemo, I would spontaneously burst into tears, a phenomenon that would only get worse as my treatments progressed. But, like a big girl I went in and took my lumps. Here's the thing. Everyone has offered support, and lots of people have truly been helpful. But at the end of the day, nobody could protect me from this treatment. Instead of Rob driving me to chemo, I wished he would kidnap me and take me somewhere else. Somewhere I could escape and the doctors couldn't find me. But that couldn't happen. So even with all of the support, love, and thoughtful gifts, I had to take all of the pokes, all of the chemo, and all of the consequences. Enduring it all was quite simply, a lonely experience.

Cancer yields endless amounts of stressful, scary, and painful moments. Sometimes it all feels insurmountable. It was hard. Very hard! To help myself move forward, each time I faced a new scary challenge or sick moment, I would remind myself that "I am good at hard things." That little mantra went through my head many times a day, and when people asked how I was getting through it, I would say it out loud.

I spent the whole day in the infusion room with Lilly, mostly trying to get some sleep. It began with the added anti-nausea drug Sustol and ended with more Neulasta fun. These bookends to my day would leave gnarly bruises and welts on the back of my arms. I never actually looked at the Sustol needle because Lilly mentioned it was large and fat. But by the way it felt going in, I had no reason to doubt her. When I finished, I went straight home to cuddle with my fur babies. I'd also like to point out that we did everything possible to keep our kids shielded from any of my scary or stressful medical stuff. We purposely did not bring them to any doctor appointments or chemo sessions. Parker was pretty relaxed about it, but Ginger was not comfortable with pokes, prods and sick people. And I didn't blame her. I wasn't comfortable either. But there was absolutely no reason to involve them in my treatments, so we didn't. They gave me hugs and cuddles when I was at home, and I tried to make fun of my bald head as much as possible.

April 9. Tuesday.

I was now scheduled to go get IV fluids every weekday for two weeks after receiving chemo. Since I really didn't like my port being accessed, my arms would get stuck with a needle each day. It was not fun, but that was my personal preference. I was in a constant state of stomach bug explosion, but fluids prevented me from having to deal with the severe side effects that come with dehydration. Being sick was bad enough. As a great gift to me, various friends pitched in to drive Ginger and Parker to and from school most days of the week. This took a huge load off of my plate. Lots of people offered lots of help, which we genuinely appreciated. But my main concern was that my children had safe rides and food to eat. Several friends contributed to make this happen. Cheryl Tyrone started a Meal Train for our family, which was absolutely awesome. We had delicious food delivered twice a week and a bunch of gift cards to use at our leisure. The only bad part about any of it was when I became too sick to send thank you cards.

April 10. Wednesday.

For the third time in just a few weeks, I had to have my head shaved. I didn't want to look like a soldier anymore, so back to Kristen's salon I went. Was I brave this time? Nay. This time she shaved the top of my head down to a #1 to match the sides. And since my remaining hair was so light blonde, I officially looked completely bald. I was an egghead, and it was jarring. One might think I would eventually get used to it, but I never did. Every single time I looked in the mirror or accidentally caught my reflection, I'd think, "Holy shit! I'm so bald." It never once looked normal to me, and I would always be taken aback. One of the better things about round #2 though, was that the spotty red rash was no longer on my face. Instead, it decided to make itself at home all over my neck and chest. For me, that felt like a win.

I also started taking extra anti-nausea meds. When I was first diagnosed, Dr. Gordan called about six different prescriptions into the pharmacy for me. I picked them up but really didn't have much of a clue as to what I was getting. I was already experiencing information overload, so I didn't do any research at the time. I believe there were two different anti-nausea meds: Phenergan and Zofran, a strong antibiotic called Cipro, and a couple of other things. None of them were thoroughly explained to me, so I didn't really know exactly how or when to take them. To complicate the matter, my father was a prescription drug addict, so I was and am utterly repulsed by drugs in general - especially the type that affects the mind. I never want to ingest anything that makes me tired or loopy because I can't stand the feeling of not being in control. So, when I looked at my bottles of anti-nausea meds, the only one I was familiar with was Phenergan. I've had it before, and it completely knocked me out. As a result, no matter how sick I was, I wouldn't touch Phenergan. While chatting with a doctor friend of mine, he mentioned that Zofran was a good choice. He said it was specifically designed for regular use and would not cause drowsiness. That sounded great, so I gave it a try. Sadly, Zofran sometimes causes headaches, and I was the lucky duck who fell into that category. Darn it! I was already having horrible headaches, that made me feel like I had bright green alien sludge rolling around under my scalp. Yes, it was bright green, and it was mean. I think the Zofran helped with nausea a bit, but to take it I had to accept an even worse headache. I couldn't win. I spent many hours each day and night curled up in beds, both home and away, with cold, wet washcloths wrapped around my head. It was old school and low tech, but it actually helped.

April 12. Thursday.

This weekend I had two banquet-style events to attend at the University of Florida. One for the Alumni awards banquet for the College of Health and Human Performance (HHP) and another for the Department of Rec Sports. It's always a thrill to go support the fantastic efforts and accomplishments of fellow Gators. These events require business or cocktail attire, and I ended up spending quite a bit of time trying to figure out which dresses would

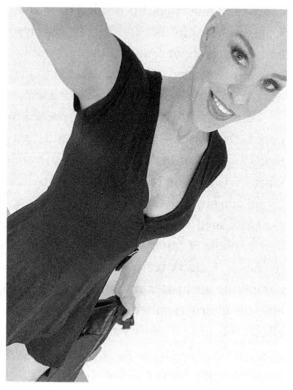

Little black dress and my little bald head.

go with my bald head. I mean, really! What was I going to wear, and which style was going to work? It practically broke my brain. And then, on the day of the HHP banquet, I finally figured it out. All of my dresses went with my bald head because they were *my* dresses. They didn't look the same way they used to, but I decided on wearing a mini black wrap dress for HHP and a short sleeveless blue dress for Rec Sports. Of course I felt like a sore thumb both nights, but I decided that standing tall and proud, pretending I felt fabulous was an important thing to do for myself. I've never stood taller, and I've never smiled bigger. I was depleted of energy and my stomach was raging, but never considered bailing on either event. They were important to me and there was no way I was going to let cancer deprive me of showing support to my Gator Nation. Point awarded to ... Fitz Koehler!

April 14. Saturday.

I was still actively searching for a solution for my nausea. Certainly, someone had to have some sort of remedy for this miserable feeling. What I found was that science says nausea itself is really non-beneficial and unproductive. No surprise there. When folks are actually compelled to expel bad stuff from their bodies, that can be a good thing because it means the body is ditching things that aren't supposed to be there. I didn't like getting sick, but at least it had a purpose. However, just sitting around feeling miserable had no benefit. My incessant tummy misery had to stop.

My research led me down the path to people singing the praises of CBD. That's the non-hallucinogenic part of the marijuana plant. I was beyond skeptical, but a lot of people swore by it. With my steady opposition to any recreational drug use, it bothered me to even be considering using anything related to marijuana. Gasp! I know some of you are rolling your eyes, and I don't care. I am who I am. I was desperate though, so I ordered some products online. I ordered pure CBD mango-flavored tinctures which didn't have any THC (the hallucinogenic part). The instructions said I was supposed to put some drops under my tongue, let them sit there for a minute, and then swallow them. They tasted disgusting and, sadly, provided no real relief. It's possible that my level of sickness was just too severe.

Eventually, I spoke to Dr. Gordan about it, and he explained that CBD can definitely help, but only when it's combined with THC. He offered to write me a prescription to see the marijuana doctor, who I would have to pay $500 in exchange for a license of use. Six weeks later I'd be able to order products myself. That sounded like a long time. Recreational marijuana use is illegal in Florida, so getting THC products the legal way would be a lengthy process. Instead, I decided to be a real rebel and grab some during my next trip to California. I know. I'm a wild and crazy girl. Any consideration of using marijuana products was far from my norm, but the nausea was unbearable, so I decided not to give a crap. In reality, I was ingesting more toxic drugs on a weekly basis than most people consume in a lifetime. What harm was some THC going to cause?

April 15. Sunday.

I think this was about the time I started completely identifying with Shrek, our favorite animated. While everyone was very complimentary about my bald head saying things like, "Ooh, it's such a great shape!" and, "Wow. You look cool like Annie Lennox!" My head shape was fine, but my skin was reacting horribly to the chemo. The rashes and bumps all over my skull were not cute, and trying to put concealer on the back of my bumpy ogre head was driving me mad. I often used two mirrors in an attempt to see what the hell I was doing, but my efforts were futile. I never once wore a hat to hide my baldness, but I did wear a hat once or twice to cover up the ogre bumps. Soon I started referring to myself as an ogre and talking like Shrek around the house and with close friends. Nobody seemed to enjoy my impersonations, though. I don't know if I enjoyed them either, but it's how I felt.

Being bald was weird in more ways than one. Sure, I looked different. Mind-bogglingly different. But it also felt very peculiar. When I was outdoors, I could feel my wee little leftover hairs blowing strangely in the wind. Sometimes they would blow one at a time, which was totally freaky. What's worse, my head was constantly cold. Chilly outdoor temperatures were a problem, but I was also forced to duck my head into my shoulders like a turtle any time I walked or sat underneath an air conditioning vent. Because of this, I kept both a trucker hat and a fuzzy hat in my bag at all times. Even during the summer. Even though I live in Florida. Backtracking a bit to aesthetic issues, I'd like to share that as a teenager, I always wondered whether the Soviet Union's President Mikhail Gorbachev knew he had that big splotchy birthmark on his head before he began balding. Had he not, that would have been quite a shock. It's because of his splotch that I always wondered if maybe I had one hiding underneath my thick blonde hair, too. Welp, I can happily report that I do not have any sort of splotchy birthmark. Unfortunately, I had something just as annoying. Once my head was shaved, I discovered that I had a long stupid suntan streak straight down the top of my head where my part was. Yep! I had a six-inch by ½ inch tan.

April 20. Friday.

Sick or not, this was a day I was going to enjoy. I had four tickets for my family to see my favorite singer of all time, Garth Brooks, at The Swamp. If you're unfamiliar with The Swamp, it's the UF football stadium, and it seats about 100,000 people. It's hard to be excited when you feel like hell, but I was. My day started off a little rough. The air was cool, so I took Piper for a walk in the morning thinking it would be good for us. Wrong. It was great for Piper, but I ended up running and heaving into my house when we were done. Apparently walking around the block was just too much for me. Scared that I might not be able to see Garth later, I decided to stay in bed until it was time to head to the show. That decision allowed me to recoup and rebound. While I'm not traditionally prone to pity parties, I felt sad as I was choosing what to wear. I was sure that all of the other girls getting ready for the concert were picking out super cute options and styling their amazing hair. Meanwhile, I was just trying to not look like a boy. It's not that I lived in total babe mode pre-cancer, but I usually walked out feeling good about myself. It wasn't a huge deal, but feeling unpretty was kind of painful. My heart hurt, and I missed the girl I used to be.

Not surprisingly, Garth was absolute perfection. He's probably one of the only individuals on Earth with enough charisma and performance power to absolutely own a massive stadium. I felt like crap, but I was still able to stand for the show and sing every word with Ginger. She's a huge Garth fan and it was so fun to have her to sing and sway with. Rob and Parker also had a good time, but in a far tamer way. While I'm obsessed with Garth's voice and energy, his song lyrics are equally dazzling. I am not the sappy type and I hate to admit this but, I definitely sat there thinking about my mortality while he sang. It was a bit painful, but that was my deal. His hit song "The Dance" gave me agonizing visions of myself crying in bed while dying at home, surrounded by family. Those thoughts were difficult, but his lyrics also comforted me as I looked back on my life. Other than cancer, I wouldn't have changed a thing about it!

To make up for the sad song, he performed a rousing cover of Tom Petty's "I Won't Back Down" toward the end of the show. As the title suggests, it's an anthem for putting up a relentless fight. And I was in the midst of mine. I'm pretty sure Garth sang it just for me.

Overall, the night was a success. I was able to enjoy the entire concert without getting sick, Garth crushed his performance, and our family was able to do something just for the fun of it. That felt like a huge win. All four of us left happy. Point awarded to, you guessed it ... the Koehlers!

April 25. Thursday.

At the crack of dawn, I boarded a plane to Monterey, California for one of the most beautiful and revered races in the entire world, the Big Sur International Marathon (BSIM). While I can honestly say that all of my races and colleagues are fabulous, the Big Sur experience is special. It's common knowledge that the location and course are mind-blowingly beautiful and posh, which is true. But, what rings most powerfully to me is the people. Many races are managed by a few rock-star individuals year-round and a larger work crew on the actual race weekend. The Big Sur Marathon Foundation comes with an elite race director, Doug Thurston, his exceptional staff, and a passionate Board of Directors, all known as "Blue Jackets." Blue Jackets are high-end event personnel who wear, you guessed it, special blue jackets! They are wholly committed to the event, the athletes, and our race production family. During race weekends, they each take on an important duty and are always easily identifiable to those who have questions or need support. Rudy introduced me to Doug in 2016, and I'm still jumping for joy that he hired me. This race family is for real, and I love to bask in their love. It's like having a bunch of cool colleagues, but also a few adoring aunts and uncles.

When I was diagnosed, I knew that my Big Sur family was horrified. They each reached out to me regularly to check in and send love. I couldn't wait to see them in person. When I arrived, I could tell they all needed to see me, too. They hugged me extra long and squeezed me extra tight. In fact, that's been kind of a thing since my diagnosis. When folks hug me, it's not the casual "great to see you" type hug. People embrace me in a way that lets me know they are grateful I'm alive. It's sweet. In fact, one of the niceties about traveling to so many places is that I get to show up and provide "proof of life." I think that when someone you love goes through something terrifying and potentially lethal, you want to get your hands on them. At least I do. So even though I felt deathly ill many times, I enjoyed being able to show up with a smile and prove to people that I was okay.

Being back at Big Sur was a blessing. Poor Doug. Like all of my race directors, he offered all sorts of relief in case I wasn't feeling well. Not only did I continuously reject his offers, but I also asked him for more obligations. Once he called to see if I wanted him to hire some sort of back-up announcer "just in case." Hell no! Of course not. Another time he called to tell me that he had a backup plan just in case I wasn't feeling up to teaching my clinic. My response was a swift, "Okay, Doug. I won't need it, but I'm glad you have it if it makes you feel better. And can I teach more than one clinic?" I believe I'm his favorite pain in the ass.

Team Noisy (Rudy and I) remains in constant motion during these busy weekends. We host the expo each day, announce the By-the-Bay 3K Saturday morning, and the marathon and shorter distance races on Sunday. I was also scheduled to teach my Strength Training for Runners clinic on Saturday afternoon, which I absolutely love doing. See, while I adore race announcing, what I really am is a fitness expert. Being able to teach a clinic that sends people home more capable and knowledgeable than they were when they arrived means everything to me. My clinics are usually packed, and my participants go on to run further, faster, and pain-free once they do what I tell them to do. They take my information and use it to PR regularly or beat the aches and pains that have been holding them back.

The one thing I did allow Doug to do for me was to have someone else host the expo on Saturday. That gave me some much-needed downtime, which worked wonders to keep me going.

April 26. Friday.

As we kicked off the weekend, Team Noisy was scheduled to meet with the local television news outlet for an interview. They were given the heads up about the race announcer with breast cancer and wanted to do a story. While I'm slightly uncomfortable being the center of attention because of sickness, I was okay with using the media to encourage folks to get annual exams and squeeze their stuff. The other thing on my mind was that Rudy has been announcing Big Sur for almost 20 years. He really deserved the recognition, so I pitched that to the reporter instead. We ended up being interviewed as Team Noisy, which was ideal. We mostly talked about what we do, how incredible BSIM is, and how much we love our athletes. When asked about my health I said, "cancer has knocked me down a bit and has taken my hair, but it hasn't taken my happy." Boom! I like it when good stuff flies out of my mouth. Our segment aired a few times over the weekend, and we were pretty pleased with it. However, they made one mistake that has yielded many laughs since. Even though we spelled and pronounced our names for the news station, they still mispronounced Rudy's last name. Instead of Novotny they pronounced it as "Novotini." Of course Rudy didn't love that error, but we decided that it made him sound like a race car driver. Vroom! Vroom!

That night, the Big Sur team hosted a VIP party for sponsors and special guests. This annual gathering is always held at Ferrante's, a fancy restaurant on the top floor of the Monterey Marriott, which has gorgeous views of the ocean and city. Most guests wear business attire, but some show up in track pants, T-shirts, and running shoes. Why? Because runners are a funny breed and, for some reason, many would find it appropriate to wear their sporty gear to a royal wedding. Perhaps they feel they must always be able to put in a few miles if a dull moment pops up. Who knows? To each their own, but I customarily enjoy the opportunity to put on a dress and be semi-lovely for an evening. Getting ready for this VIP party was challenging, though. I remember putting on my makeup and short black wrap dress and not really loving it. That bald head of mine was becoming a real nuisance. I used to feel kind of pretty when I got all dolled up, but this time I felt like an ogre in a dress. But staying back and wallowing in self-pity was not an option, so I put on my proverbial "big girl panties" and made the choice to fake it. Fake confidence. Fake joy. Fake health. I stood there in my hotel bathroom and took a giant deep breath before Rudy grabbed me to go. I remember staring into the mirror thinking, "How the hell did I get here?" It didn't matter. This is where I was, this is what I looked like, and the show had to go on. And on it went.

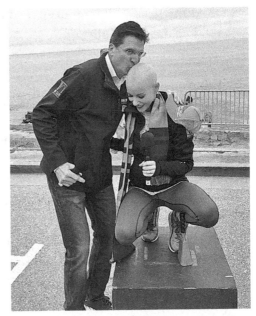

Head kisses from BSIM race director Doug Thurston

When I got to the party, I decided to hold my chin up higher than ever and smile like absolutely nothing was wrong. It was hard, but I had previously lived by the motto "Fake it till you make it" and "Never let 'em see you sweat." This was an unusual circumstance, but the strategy was the same. The party was full of happy faces and friendly conversation, and my performance allowed me to blend right in.

The next day, a gaggle of women approached me to gush over my look from the party. Apparently they thought I was a model who had chosen to go bald for shock value or style value or something like that. They told me they were mesmerized by me and were so envious of my confidence! I don't share this because I believe I'm a hot dish or that anyone has any real reason to believe I'm any sort of supermodel. But they were genuinely shocked when I told them that I was undergoing chemo for breast cancer. They hadn't viewed me as an insecure or sick chick because that's not what I projected. Booyah! Lesson learned. Even though pretending to be fabulous was a challenge, the greatest thing I could do was hold my head high and keep a smile on my face. Confidence, even when faked, is powerful stuff.

April 27. Saturday.

4:30 a.m. came pretty fast as I woke up and leapt into the shower. Showers were quick and easy these days, as I had no hair to wash, dry, or style. Neat! What wasn't neat was my shock when I peered into the mirror for the first time. My pale gray-blue eyes had turned *navy!* What? Tracey didn't tell me that was a possible side effect of chemo. None of the informative cancer brochures mentioned anything of the sort. Holy hell! What happened to my eyes? I was both stunned and angry. But I continued to get ready because, you know, thousands of people were literally waiting for me. My eyes didn't feel bad, nor had my vision been altered, but I was certainly thrown for a loop. Was it all in my head? No. My eyes were definitely 50 shades darker than they had been the day before. This was confirmed when Rudy came to my room to pick me up and instantly noticed the change. Since nothing seemed to dramatically change with

my health, I moved on with my day with a big stupid question mark over my head. Eventually, my eyes faded from navy to royal blue, but they still haven't gone back to the pale gray-blue I started out with. Weird.

Announcing the By-the-Bay 3K with Rudy was a delectable way to kick off our races. The event focuses on school children and their families, and had more than 5,000 people in attendance. He hosted the main stage, while I announced the start and finish line. Getting to spend time with the kids and their active parents just fills my

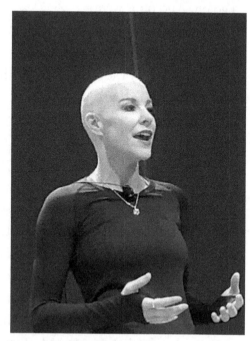

Teaching my clinic.
Photo by Dianne Chan

heart with the good stuff. I've functioned on adrenaline all year, and I can promise you this — if I'm at a race full of kids, I feel nothing but elation. We were all pretty cold, and my nose never stopped running, but it was a fantastic morning. The year before I had taken on the duty of warming everyone up with a choreographed dance, I called "The Big Sur Stomp." I just wasn't up to that level of energy this time, so I skipped it. No one asked me to do it, and I didn't offer. I'm sure it was missed, but I'll definitely bring it back when my energy returns.

Next up for the afternoon was my Strength Training for Runners clinic. I was very eager to teach it, but also slightly leery. Chemo brain is a real thing, and I had begun to forget some of the finer points in life. I never struggled with major concepts, but I had been foggy on names, details, and words. Yes, I was struggling to find words, which isn't a positive development for a professional speaker. I never speak with a script. I just teach what I know, and I do it with ease. My presentations are entertaining, engaging, and thorough as heck. Folks leave with information that has the opportunity to change their lives. I was hoping that this slightly dulled version of myself could keep up with full-blown Fitz Koehler. That girl could do incredible things.

I took the big stage of the Monterey Conference Center and greeted my sizable audience. Since there was a big poster of me out front with my long fabulous hair, I decided to address the elephant in the room. Because my audience didn't show up to hear about me I kept it brief. I took my hat off to expose my very bald head and gave them the 90-second spiel. "Clean mammogram in December, found a lump in February, life is tricky right now, but I'm curable. Everyone needs to squeeze their stuff because early detection saves lives." The end. My delivery was light and breezy, and I was happy to move on. The rest of my clinic went fantastic, and I was able to perform exactly as I'd hoped, except for losing two words. Yep. I had two moments mid-presentation, where I just couldn't pull up the word I was looking for. Fortunately, when I described what I wanted to say, my audience helped me come up with "plantar fasciitis" and, well, I still can't remember the other one. Chemo brain *is* real.

When ending my presentations, I always share that I'll clear the stage for the next presenter and remain available nearby in case anyone wants to chat. Practically everyone stuck around. I stood outside the room with a line a mile long, full of sweet people who wanted to ask questions, take pics, or simply wish me well. More often than not, I end up with a ton of people who want to talk or take pics post-presentation, but this crew was unique. Again, these are the type of hugs and sweetness one only experiences when people are genuinely feeling grateful that you're alive. I'm a lucky lady. Of note, Buffy Harrison brought me a fun "F*** Cancer" trucker hat, which I love. We took a cute picture in our hats, flipping the bird and shared it proudly on social media. And Christie Marriott stuck around to visit and share her personal experience with breast cancer. Our time together was enjoyable and encouraging. I'm pretty sure I was in my bed and unconscious by 6 p.m.

April 28. Sunday.

The Big Sur International Marathon is a big deal. Not only because it's one of the most notable race weekends in the world, but also because it's pretty complicated logistically. We put on five different races with four different start lines and one grand finish line. Besides the full marathon, we have a 21-miler, an 11-miler, a 12K, a 5K, and a relay race. Before I go any further, I should tell you a little bit about the full marathon course and why it's on almost every Top Ten Marathon list in the world. The 26.2-mile journey takes you through the most stunning portions of scenic Highway 1, where the ocean crashes into an endless row of rocky cliffs. The elevation changes are diverse, exhilarating, and challenging as hell. Climbing "Hurricane Point" with a headwind provided by the ocean, for example, is one of the obstacles that runners both lose sleep over and dream about during the months leading up to their race. They also get to sightsee on foot as they tour Pfeiffer Big Sur State Park, farmlands, redwood trees, and the Point Sur Lighthouse. Athletes have the unique opportunity to cross the famous Bixby Creek Bridge on foot, which can only be done on race day. At the end of that bridge, they are treated to music by classical pianist Michael Martinez (complete with tuxedo and tails), which adds an elegant touch. Earning an entry into this event is a privilege and one that our runners' remember forever.

Rudy started his morning 26.2-miles down the road from me at Big Sur Station to launch the full marathon, while I went straight to the finish line. The finish line is also the start line of the 12K and 5K, and it's our other top priority stage. Several board members volunteer to start the 21-miler and the 11-miler. Launching the 5K and 12K was a blast because our runners were in high spirits. They were excited about their races, but I think they were equally thrilled that they were not about to run 26.2 miles. Not that those doing the longer distance races weren't in for a treat, but the people I was dealing with did not have nearly as daunting an experience in their immediate future. They were just out for a cool Sunday morning spin around a beautiful town. Once I yelled "GO", I stayed in place so 100% of our athletes would receive a champion's welcome when they were done. Eventually, Rudy made it to the finish line to join me, but it took him a couple of hours to get there by car after he yelled "GO" for the full marathoners.

With fatigue and nausea trying to take me down, I was relieved that my athletes gave me the go-go juice I needed to work at full throttle. The finish line was rocking all day as the crowds were huge, and the runners were elated to have conquered Big Sur. Rudy and I just danced our day away as we poured huge amounts of love on our runners. And, while we had noisy fun on our stage, a dozen of our Blue Jackets showed up to check on us. They had no obligation to do so, but this is just the type of thoughtful people they are. I felt their love from the moment I arrived until the moment I left. And I hope they felt mine too. In the middle of hell, Big Sur allowed me to experience pure joy. That evening, I packed up and headed to the airport for my red-eye flight home, where I would get to chemo at 10:15 a.m.

April 29. Monday.

Of course, I couldn't sleep at all on the plane ride from San Jose to Atlanta. And of course, my sick tummy was a jerk all night long. I don't write about it often, but for the record, my stomach wreaked havoc on me every single day for five solid months. Every morning I woke up the same way a frat boy with a tequila hangover wakes up. So, while I was at airports, terminals, start lines, finish lines, clinics, and important events with my kids, I was managing the likes of a tequila hangover. Since my cancer was a quickly replicating kind, the chemo I was given attacked all quickly replicating cells in my body. My hair, nails, and entire digestive system fell into this category. From my mouth on out, it felt like my innards were being put through a cheese grater. And in a sense they were. The imagery is awful, but that was my reality. My taste buds, throat, stomach, and more were literally being destroyed and I felt every bit of it. Waaaah!

Even though I didn't sleep much during the flight, I actually felt less bothered than usual. I knew that once I got to chemo, Lilly would give me a big bag of Benadryl, and I would probably pass out for most of the day. My flight landed in Gainesville at 9:30 a.m. and my appointment with Dr. Gordan, followed by chemo, was at 10:15 a.m. Seamless. But, one of the bummer details about having to go straight from the plane to chemo was that I couldn't stop home to see Piper and Handy. It's funny, I definitely miss my humans when I'm gone, but technology allows me to call or FaceTime with them, which really takes the edge off. But when it comes to my pets, I'm pretty much completely cut off since they're terrible on the phone. Seeing tons of other dogs at the races made me miss mine so much more. Plus everyone always asked about my adorable duck, who was basically social media famous. I really would have liked to pop in for some feathered and furry love that morning, but straight to chemo I went. I felt and looked like hell, but I was able to sleep in my chemo recliner, and that was a simple gift for this very tired race announcer.

At about 5:00 p.m., I was awoken with taps on my shoulder by someone I wasn't expecting to see. It was Parker saying, "Hey Mom!" While I was excited to see his sweet face, I was confused because Rob and I had decided not to bring the kids to any of my appointments. It was weird, but I was super groggy and thought that maybe he just wanted to come to pick me up since I'd been out of town for a handful of days. Once my Neulasta was attached, and I was able to leave, we headed out into the giant lobby of the cancer center. Again, I was surprised to see Ginger.

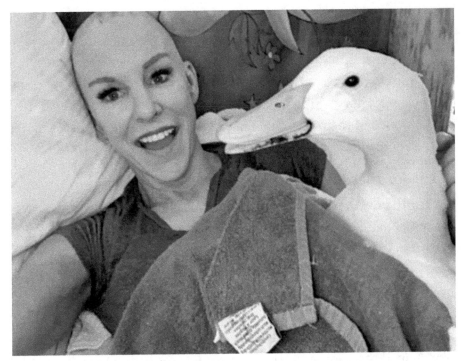

Handy made me laugh nonstop. #BestDuckEver

She greeted me with a sweet hug, and then Rob asked me to sit down. I knew that his "Sit down" was code for "Something terrible has happened." When I sat down, poor Rob said, "It's Handy." Gut punch and instant heartbreak. I sobbed so hard.

Not once through this cancer nightmare had I thought "This isn't fair" or "Why me?" Not once! But this was just the cruelest kick in the teeth. Losing Handy was mean. She brought so much joy, fun, and love to my momentarily-harrowing life. When I felt like hell, she cuddled up in my arms for a nap or made me laugh with her sassy quacks. She gave me something to look forward to, and boy did I look forward to being with her. She was the ultimate distraction from cancer and sickness; I loved her so much and needed her so badly. It was crushing. Occasionally, I still break down because I miss her. Ugh. The good news is that she died naturally. Nothing harmful happened to her. She was just resting next to her Ducky Dream House when she passed peacefully. Poor Rob was panicked over the effect her death would have on me. When we got home, I instantly went out back to see her. Rob put my sweet, bright white, love-bomb duck in my arms, and I sat with her for a couple of hours. After singing the "Rubber Ducky" song to her one last time, I asked him to take us to the farm where she came from so that we could bury her. Of course, John and Cheryl Tyrone allowed that. She's buried in the woods of their property. I'm pretty sure I will miss that duck for the rest of my life.

April 30. Tuesday.

For the next few months, my days at home looked the same. I was crazy sick, and if I wasn't at some sort of medical appointment, I was curled up in bed. I needed rest desperately and my functionality was severely diminished. I wasn't cooking, cleaning, driving my kids around, exercising, returning many emails, socializing, or doing much of anything else. Not only was I resting because my body needed me to, but also because I was constantly in a state of resting up before my next work trip. If there was a timelapse camera on my bedroom ceiling, you'd see a constant stream of pictures of Piper and me twisted up together in various formations. Sweet dog, she spent every ounce of energy she had taking care of me. It was incredible to see her spring into action once I was diagnosed. I am 100% positive that she knew I was sick and needed her. She never left my side and I was grateful for her loyalty. If I went to the bathroom, she went to the bathroom. If I went to the couch, she went with me. We would often lie in bed together all day. Her warm little body felt like heaven on earth and I took hundreds of naps with my head on her tushy. While I felt guilty for burdening my humans with relentless sickness, sadness, and a lack of productivity, Piper was my go-to for long days of rest sans guilt. I lost my ability to take her out for walks sometime in April and felt incredibly guilty about that. Before cancer and chemo, we were constantly playing or walking, but all of that had come to a halt. Rob, Ginger, and Parker would walk her, but not as frequently as I did. I promised her every day that I would make sure she had all of the walks, playtime, and love that she could handle once I was feeling better. I've been keeping that promise.

My amazing human caretaker was Rob. He drove me to all of my doctor appointments, chemo appointments, scans, and everything in between. When I was frail and sickly, he walked slowly with me while holding me up so I wouldn't fall down. He made sure I had food, wash-cloths for the painful green alien sludge in my head, and anything else I needed. I won't harp on that, but it's imperative that you know how much he did. If I was at home, he was doting on me. And he also carried the type of load a single parent would have. He did all of the cooking, cleaning, driving, yardwork, shopping, homework help, and more. We were all lucky to have him.

Fitzness Log

Since my second round of chemo was pushed back I had an extra week before being poisoned again. That gave me a sliver of time to start exercising again. It was rewarding to be able to take Piper on walks and do strength training at the gym. I feel like the best version of myself when I have a weight in my hand. I love being physically strong and adore the process of making muscles. For those reasons, I pursue that element of fitness training most aggressively. On the day before chemo #2, I even felt well enough to do some running on a treadmill. I wasn't breaking any records with my pace, but it still felt wonderful to do something so vigorous. It was also the first time I'd ever gone running without having to manage a ponytail! Running bald was convenient, but strange. Is this how men live? Very interesting!

Chemo #2 knocked me out of exercising for the next two weeks. But in my third week, I was able to go back to the gym. My quads were super weak and sore from chemo, but the rest of me was happy to be chal-lenged. I was not killing it by any means, instead, I was going through my normal strength training routine at about 50% of what I used to do. And I was fine with that. I also allotted a ton of time to stretching be-cause my poor muscles were incredibly tight.

Chapter 5

Blind Faith in Myself

May 1. Wednesday.

This was another fun day. #NotReally. On my way to the cancer center to get IV fluids, I stopped by the little coffee shop in the giant lobby. I was wearing a black jacket and a trucker hat because it was chilly outside. As I approached the guy behind the counter, he looked at me and greeted me with, "Hey Buddy, what can I get you? Oh! You're a ma'am! Sorry!" I instantly burst into tears. Big tears. I have never in my life been confused for a man, and there it was. Bald and pale and ogre-like, it happened. Poor guy. I don't blame him for the confusion because I didn't look very feminine at the moment. But sadly for both of us, I didn't have my usual strength and ability to laugh it off and say, "It's no big deal." Instead, I just walked off toward the infusion room. Sobbing uncontrollably.

When I approached Shirley's check-in desk, she asked why I was crying and I told her what happened. She did her best to comfort me, but I was inconsolable. I felt terrible that I was making her feel so bad, but I couldn't stop my waterworks. I loved looking like a girl, and this stung. Big time. From that day on, every time I checked in with Shirley, she would greet me with a "Hi, beautiful" or "Hey, gorgeous." She went overboard to try and undo the damage the coffee shop guy had done. That's actually one of the nice things about going through cancer treatment. Almost everyone I know has made an overt effort to be extra kind. And it's never gone unappreciated. Not once. But from that day forward, I made sure to never leave the house without bright lipstick.

May 3. Friday.

Itinerary:

- May 3: Fly to Orange County, California
- May 4: Kids Run the OC, OC 5k
- May 5: OC Marathon and Half Marathon
- May 9: Fly to Little Rock, Arkansas
- May 10: DC Wonder Woman Run Expo
- May 11: DC Wonder Woman Run 10K and 5K, Fly to Detroit, Michigan
- May 12: Ann Arbor Goddess 5K, 1-Mile, and Kid Races, Fly Home

It was 4:30 a.m. and four days after chemo #3. I was boarding a plane to California, to start what would be an 11-day trip, announcing in three different states. Once again, Rob walked me up to TSA asking me how I was going to do this, and again I stared blankly, shrugged my shoulders, and replied "I just will." That's kind of been my motto, and it's worked pretty well so far. Up first, I was headed back to announce the OC Marathon Weekend for the sixth time. This was one of my most demanding events of the year, and since I was arriving four days post-chemo, I had FaceTimed race director, Gary Kutscher, a few weeks prior with what may have qualified as his weirdest request ever. "Hey, Gary. Chemo has been kind of mean and makes me pretty sick. I'm going to be able to work, but can you help me get some IV fluids while I'm there?" Poor guy. I could see the surprise on his sweet smiling face as he said, "Sure! I'll figure that out." And he did. He arranged a bit of a trade with a local business called The Hydration Room. In exchange for a booth at his Expo, they hooked me up with free saline a couple of times that weekend. Dehydration was a huge problem that would have definitely prevented me from performing well over the weekend, so the arrangement made all of the difference.

One of the loveliest gestures of the entire year happened during my first flight of the day. Now, it's only a 50-minute flight, so it's actually hard for anything significant to happen in transit. Luckily for me, kindness doesn't require much time. When I took my seat in row five or so, the flight attendant made a beeline for me to see if I needed anything. I wasn't in first class, and if I were, this would make complete sense. But I was in Delta Comfort, which is somewhere between coach and first class as far as luxuries go. You get a little bit more wiggle room and sometimes better snacks, but you do not get food and beverage service before the flight takes off. Still, this compassionate man was coming to check on the glossy-eyed bald chick. I wasn't wearing any pink ribbons or any other identifying items that told the world I had cancer. He just knew. I appreciated his effort, especially because I felt a little like death warmed over that morning, but the only things that could actually help me were things he couldn't provide. I graciously thanked him and told him I'd be okay.

Once our flight took off, he walked by with the beverage cart and again asked if I needed anything. While I didn't actually like any of the snacks available, I agreed to a package of cookies because my tummy was a bit rumbly and I thought some food might help. I just needed a little something to hold me over until I arrived in Atlanta. I only asked for one, but he gave me three. Three bags of cookies I didn't really like, but I appreciated the gesture. And then he promised he'd be back with more if there were any left. After he served the whole plane and walked back up to the front with his cart, he paused next to me and proceeded to plop about 10 packages of cookies on my tray table! It was so cute and sweet. All I can imagine is this guy probably lost someone very dear to cancer. I could tell that he just desperately needed to care for me, so I accepted those cookies, and thanked him with a smile. He took it just a step further as I was walking off the plane. As I reached the exit, he reached out, put something in my hand , and said, "I'm rooting for you." I thanked him again, continued walking, and then opened my hand to find a rock! A simple but pretty, smooth, brown, and gray marbled rock. I'm guessing it was his lucky rock. I wanted to run back and give him a big "thank you" hug, but the flow of other passengers prevented me from making that move. While I have not enjoyed cancer nor the treatment for it, I really have been delighted by the constant gestures of goodwill toward me because of it. That lucky rock still sits on my nightstand and it makes me smile all the time.

When I landed in the OC, Rudy picked me up from the airport and we drove straight to The Hydration Room. I remember collapsing my head down on his armrest. I was physically exhausted and mentally drained from having to act like a functioning human all day. It was nice to have no responsibilities for at least a few minutes until we arrived for my IV fluids. It had only been four days since chemo, and I was experiencing the height of my chemo-induced misery. A 9-hour travel day wasn't a fun way to recover. However, nothing in the world was going to keep me away from the OC Marathon Weekend. I was super sick, but also thrilled to be in Newport Beach, and legitimately eager to get to work.

The Hydration Room was kind of like a nail salon, but with IVs instead of polish. Even though I was so pleased that I could get IV fluids without the full drama, expense, and ordeal of a hospital, I still found the concept of an IV salon a little odd. The idea that regular non-sick people would volunteer and even pay to be injected with fluids seemed weird. It's seriously not something I would ever do outside of a medical crisis, but apparently, lots of people are into it. The second thing that I questioned was the professional capabilities of the people at these spas. Who in the world worked at a place like this?

Well, when I arrived, I asked. It turned out that the folks hooking up IVs were actual nurses who did this as a side gig. In fact, one of the women who treated me was an oncology nurse. She worked with cancer patients all the time, which was really comforting. When I asked if she had any special tricks for beating nausea, we ended up having a long conversation about CBD products. I told her I'd bought some and they weren't really helping. Like Dr. Gordan, she said that I needed to add the THC component for success and recommended a local place where I could buy some. Since it's something I had been contemplating anyway, I planned to use her referral after the races concluded. Taking anything new or mind-altering on a race weekend was a no-go. When I was done, I took an Uber to my hotel, where I was finally able to collapse and sleep for the night with a cold washcloth on my head full of green alien sludge.

May 4. Saturday.

Gary and his sidekick, Kelsey Beall, do an extraordinary job with the OC Marathon. It has a cool beach party vibe, and everyone shows up extra happy. Our *Kids Run the OC* event involves about 10,000 kids ages three to 12 and their coaches. As usual, stepping on to my stage transformed my illness into awesomeness. Zing! I was juiced up and fully charged. I announced the kids' races for about four hours and enjoyed every moment of it. Rudy hosted the coinciding festival but popped in to check on me here and there. I launched about nine different age-specific races that morning, which meant that after giving the kids their pre-race instructions and pumping them all up, I yelled "go" nine different times. If you don't know, yelling "go" (in a very big way) is very big fun.

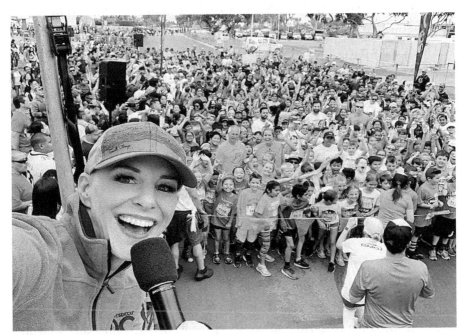

Kids Run the OC start line.

I also welcomed them all through the finish line. When our final kid conquered the one-mile course, I borrowed Rudy's car to go get more IV fluids. Then I took a little nap in his car before returning to announce the OC 5K.

Rudy lives in Southern California and I consider it my home-base for races, so this weekend felt a bit like a class reunion. It was packed with Team Noisy friends and we relished getting to see so many people we care about. Of course, the sweetness generated toward me was over-the-top. Runners came with concern, kindness, and gifts. Lots of thoughtful gifts. Whenever Rudy declared that he felt like chopped liver, I'd simply remind him that if he wanted a little more attention, all he needed was a little bit of cancer. After that he continuously chose to be chopped liver. The OC 5K was a blast and a great way to close out the day. We did lots and lots of talking and thoroughly enjoyed every minute of it. After grabbing some dirt-covered pasta for dinner, I planted my butt in bed as quickly as possible in order to prepare for another 4 a.m. wake-up call.

May 5. Sunday.

Long races tend to start absurdly early so that runners can finish up before the heat becomes oppressive, and so roads are only closed during the least busy part of the day. It's a smart formula for success. It's unpleasant to get up so early sometimes, but it's not a huge sacrifice, considering how much I love announcing. The start line for the OC Marathon and Half Marathon lies on a gorgeous palm tree-lined road surrounding the fancy pants mall in Newport Beach called Fashion Island. Stepping onto this particular start line stage each year is always special to me. I love that it was the first race that I ever announced. I love Gary and Kelsey. And I delight in the endless stream of friends that pop in for a hug. At 4:45 a.m., Rudy and I started the show. We played fun music, bantered, provided pre-race instructions, plugged sponsors, blah, blah, blah. We always laugh with our runners so much that you'd think we were all just hanging out in our kitchens chatting.

At 5:30 a.m., we launched the marathon. When our 1,600 athletes took off for their 26.2-mile adventure, we went back into our welcome spiel for the athletes who were running the half marathon, which was scheduled to start at 6:15 am. The half marathon was much larger with about 7,000 participants, so we broke them up into smaller starting groups called corrals. Many races do this to prevent log jams out on the course. Starting 1,000 people every five minutes often creates just enough space in between athletes so that they can run or walk at a comfortable pace without too much congestion. As it happens every year, Rudy and I launched the first half marathon corral together, and then he left to drive to the finish line with Gary. That left me alone to party and play with the remaining corrals of half marathoners, which meant about six more giant "go's" for me.

Here's something you should know. When we start races, we do so in a very BIG way. We whip our athletes into a legit frenzy, and we yell "GO" in a way that's worthy of the special races we preside over. We never do a countdown, as they're almost always lame and highly anti-climatic. And, whenever possible, we do not use air horns, which make one of the least-exciting and most-annoying sounds on the planet. We specialize in big energy and big fun. Countdowns are not fun. Air horns are not fun. Our "Runners, Set, GOOOO!" is power-packed with excitement and serves as the pressure release valve once our athletes are hyped up and ready to run. And here's the other thing you should know about the way we do things. It all started with Rudy Novotny, who has been announcing races for 30ish years. While I bring incredible energy, content, and style to the announcer stage, he's been doing it forever, has a big booming voice, and is massively charismatic. He's my favorite race announcer and I'm grateful he has shared so many stages with me. When I yell "GO," I never try to copy him per se, because I could never belt it out the way he does with *that voice*. However, with my solid and strong lady-voice, I do a pretty fine job as well.

Being with these corrals isn't just about the "GO." It's about connecting with them and making their personal moments at the start line as special as possible. While I completely respect and admire the speedsters up in the front corrals, I find that the further back we go the more fun the people are. The OC corrals look more like parties than people waiting to begin a race. We dance, jump, sing, laugh, and do more than race. Luck-

ily I'm pretty sure zero people knew that I felt like death
several hours earlier. Why?
Because I was plugged in,
turned on, and running off
of runner-generated go-go
juice. As usual, once I yelled
"GO" for the last time and
the final runners crossed the
start line, I instantly became
sad that they were gone.

Within minutes, I
jumped into Kelsey's car and
we headed to the finish line.
Fifteen minutes later, I was
back on stage with Rudy,
where we engaged and en-
tertained the spectators until
the runners started arriving.

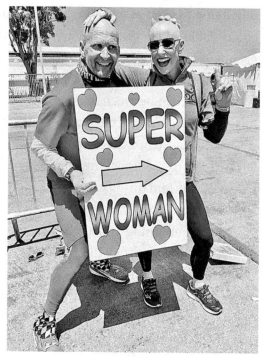

With the "Jester" of running,
Ed Ettinghausen.

My incredible race playlist kept everyone invigorated for hours, and we
loved being the first to personally, and publicly, congratulate 9,000 runners as they conquered their 13.1 or 26.2-mile courses.

Throughout the day I had Rudy in my ear telling me to take a break,
which is something he does at every race. Sometimes I find it hilarious
and other times I find it annoying. He's been doing it for years, and I
always respond with, "No!" Especially at OC, because we have so many
friends on the course and I hate missing any of their finishes. It's become
a game of sorts that makes both of us cranky. But this time I'm pretty
sure Rudy was telling me to take a break because he was genuinely concerned for me. But cancer or no cancer, I was going to work at 100%. I
did, on occasion, run into the VIP tent to grab food, but only because
Rudy and I were on the mic until about 3 p.m. It was a long, exciting,
and busy day, and I felt mostly great the whole time. But the second we
said good-bye, I could feel my body starting to shut down. If you listened

closely, you probably could have heard my body making noises as if my internal battery died. It was early, but I was ready for bed. I had definitely overdone it, and was starting to feel every ounce of sickness that I'd been able to tamp down during the weekend.

May 6. Monday.

This was the start of a very long and tricky week. I had to fly to Little Rock, Arkansas, on Thursday to announce the DC Wonder Woman Run Series on Friday and Saturday. Then I had to fly to Detroit, Michigan, on Saturday evening to host the Ann Arbor Goddess 5K on Sunday morning. So I decided to hunker down in Rudy's cozy guest room instead of returning home to Florida. This allowed me to skip a full day of California to Florida travel and instead stay in a place where I had zero obligations. It was going to be an 11-day gauntlet, and I thought, "If I can announce these seven races in three different states, I win!" Full-force Fitz Koehler would have giddily bounced through it all. Chemo Fitz Koehler was excited, but also anxiously hoping everything would go her way.

Sadly, I woke up in my hotel room with zero voice. Zero. I wasn't hoarse or raspy; I was mute. Uh-oh. My guess is that the combination of chemo's effect on my throat and a nonstop weekend of big talking with those 17 big "GO's" was just too much. Being completely silent is never good for someone who speaks for a living. I was also at about 0% energy and my stomach was a mess. I had definitely overdone it. Before Rudy drove us to his home in San Diego, he was going to take me to the shop the oncology nurse recommended. I haven't mentioned this before, but Rudy is 33 years clean and sober. This situation could have possibly made me the worst person in the world or him the best person in the world. But he was 100% eager to help, and I wasn't too worried that a little stop at this shop would risk him ruining his extraordinary three decades of sobriety.

When we arrived in the industrial area, we were both pretty surprised. It wasn't the gross little head shop that we had imagined at all. Instead, the store was big, clean, and high tech with heavily armed security guards throughout. I signed in on an iPad and we relaxed in the lobby before my name was called to go into the showroom. Since I was voiceless, Rudy had to do all of the talking for me. When the 20-something big bearded man greeted us, he was surprisingly professional. Rudy informed him that I had breast cancer and that I was looking to get help with my nausea, without getting high. He recommended tinctures, which had a 1:10 ratio of THC to CBD. There were far stronger options available, but I took his advice and paid $100 cash for the two tiny bottles I called "pot drops." I was now the pothead on Team Noisy, which made us laugh even more. Now, here's the deal: I took them, but they never really had a major impact on my nausea. Maybe the stuff I got wasn't strong enough, or maybe I was just too sick for help. But I definitely gave them a try. A few months later, I ended up getting THC gummy worms that were a bit stronger. They eased my tummy slightly, but I found that they were more useful for helping me fall asleep.

After our big drug deal, we headed to Rudy's house, and I proceeded to lie down, watch TV, and sleep for the next four days. I wasn't quick to recover, and I never really felt anything that resembled good. It was a price I was happy to pay for the career that I loved, but three rounds of chemo in, I was feeling like hell. I was warned that chemo would be cumulative, meaning that I would feel worse and be slower to recover after each infusion. That was coming true. The main concern I was having, though, was my lack of sound. I had to announce two fantastic events in Arkansas and Michigan in a few days and I needed to be able to speak. I was frustrated and felt like Ariel, The Little Mermaid, when she had her voice snatched by Ursula. I was fully committed to not speaking a word and letting my vocal cords rest, but I'd wake up each morning still mute. On Wednesday morning, I emailed Dr. Gordan begging for help. He quickly called in a prescription for steroids, which are known to help with severe laryngitis. An hour later, I had them in my hand. The race was on to get my voice back before Friday morning. I did not panic, but I was definitely concerned. I drank lots of water, remained super silent, took my steroids, and hoped a whole lot. I even stayed silent when trying to communicate with my kids. Parker doesn't like to chat on the phone too much, so he was happy to exchange texts. Ginger loves to talk a lot though. In order to keep her satisfied, we would FaceTime every day, and she would talk, talk, talk, and I would respond with facial or hand gestures. Silly at times, but it worked. How lucky am I to have a teenage daughter who wants to discuss everything?

On Thursday morning, Rudy drove me to the San Diego Airport to ship me off to Little Rock, still with no voice. Now it was his turn to ask me how I was going to do it. I just shrugged my shoulders and let him know that "I just would." Call it blind faith, but I have always seemed to pull things off no matter what, so I trusted that everything would work out. I suppose if I have to have blind faith in anyone, it might as well be in me, right?

As Murphy's Law would have it, my first flight was delayed, which made me miss my connecting flight from Atlanta to Little Rock. Then my second flight was delayed due to foul weather, and I didn't arrive in Little Rock until almost 1 a.m. My energy tank was empty, and I was still unable to generate any sound. I was desperate to get to my hotel room, where our event team had left a humidifier for me. I hadn't told my race director, Beth Salinger, that I was completely mute because I didn't want to worry her. Instead, I told a white lie, claiming I had caught a little cough and sore throat from someone at OC.

When my plane landed, I quickly grabbed my luggage and opened up the Uber app to catch a ride. For the first time ever, Uber told me that there were zero drivers working in the area at the time. What? No drivers? Nope. None. I looked for taxis, and there weren't any of those either. Now I was in Little Rock, AR with no Uber, no taxis, no rental car, and no voice. Shit! Life kind of sucked at that moment. I had to laugh, though, because the absurdity of it all was just too much. I had considered finding an airport police officer for help, but eventually decided to download the Lyft app instead. Thankfully, there was one driver in the area, and she was all mine. It took her about 20 minutes to arrive and pick up my lonely last-girl-in-the-airport butt, but I can't tell you how grateful I was to see her. On the way to my hotel, she played really vulgar rap music "n-word this, b-word that" and she smacked her lips while chewing gum like a cow. But did I care? Nope! I was just grateful to be going toward a bed. Hallelujah, for me. Big tip for her.

When I finally arrived at the hotel, the humidifier was waiting at the front desk. I placed it right on top of my nightstand, so the humidity would be force-fed into my face as I slept, and hopefully work its miracles. I definitely needed some.

May 10. Friday.

I woke up groggy yet grateful that I didn't have to be at the expo until noon. It was cold and rainy outside, so our team had moved our expo and finish line festival indoors for the weekend. Groggy as I was, I had one thing on my mind. My voice. I actually waited a little while to test it, as if an extra 30 minutes of silence would make a difference, but then it happened. I opened up my mouth and said, "hello." It was hoarse and scratchy, but it was SOUND! My voice was definitely not what it was supposed to be, but it existed, and I could work with that. I had a huge smile on my face as I put on my Wonder Woman tutu. I needed these wins. Cancer stunk, and chemo was trying to kill me (while saving me), so I just needed the world to allow me to do the work that I loved. If my cancer treatment had made me miss this race, I would have been helpless, and that is something I did not want to be. I kept my talking to a minimum while hosting the expo, so I'd be good for the next two days of actual race announcing. I still wasn't out of the woods, so as soon as the expo was over, I hurried back to my hotel room to pass out and inhale the humidifier.

May 11. Saturday.

I woke up with a voice again. Outstanding! Things were looking good. I arrived at the indoor venue around 6 a.m. for our pre-race gathering, and the runners started filling the place up. It was a dark and rainy day, so it was awesome to be inside for a while. This was actually my first DC Wonder Woman Run Series race since my diagnosis. There were two others held a month prior, but someone else covered them since I was already committed to announcing the Los Angeles and Big Sur Marathons. I hate that I can't be in two places at once. So rude!

Nonetheless. I hadn't announced a DC Wonder Woman Run Series race since the fall and I really missed it. I missed our team, our runners, our vibe, and Wonder Woman. Like all of my races, the DC Wonder Woman Run Series is a standout and special for a variety of reasons. Like for many of us, she was my childhood hero. I obsessively watched the Linda Carter TV show. I considered my Wonder Woman Underoos my "uniform" and wore them as much as possible. I also once dressed up as Wonder Woman for Halloween in that horrible plastic costume. The one with the plastic mask, which was affixed to my face with a constantly-breaking and snapping rubber band. When I was approached about hosting this event series, I definitely reverted back to being a giddy five-year-old. The answer wasn't "Yes." It was "Hell yes!"

When I contacted the creator and owner of this series, Mark Knutson, to share my diagnosis, he offered me the opportunity to talk to our athletes about it. And this morning, I decided to do so. With a couple thousand athletes and their supporters gathered, I took to the stage and took off my hat. I assure you; nothing silences a room faster than the revelation that your bouncy, bubbly race announcer is (gasp) bald. With the music down super low, I quickly shared my story. "On December 28th, I had a clean mammogram. Then on February 21st I found a lump. I have breast cancer. It's not been fun, but because of my self-exam, and extraordinary science, there is a light at the end of the tunnel. While you're all already making efforts to improve your health by participating in athletic adventures like these DC Wonder Woman Run Series races, you need to go further. Watch what you put in your mouth, get enough sleep, get your annual exams, and SQUEEZE YOUR STUFF! The crowd went wild. Not only do you need to squeeze your own stuff, but you should squeeze your romantic partner's stuff too. Be proactive. Pause taking care of everyone else, and start taking some time for yourselves instead. From here on out, set an alarm on your phone for those self-exams every Wednesday morning at 7 a.m. You may just save your own life." That's a brief synopsis of my presentation, and it's the one I decided to stick with from that point on. Clear and concise with actionable directions for people to move forward with. Oh, and my bald head turned out to be a very powerful tool for me. Did I like it? No way. Was it a profound way to get folks to pay attention? Absolutely.

After the indoor morning fun with our Wonder Woman trivia and costume contest, we moved things outside to the start line. Nobody complained about the yucky weather. Runners and walkers are cool like that. Instead, they danced in their ponchos and garbage bags celebrating Wonder Woman until Linda Carter (pre-recorded and displayed on the big screen) and I yelled, "GO!" Now, I normally adore commanding this vibrant circus of a sport. Having Wonder Woman at my side is just icing on the cake. I'll probably get lashed with a wet noodle or something for this, but our Wonder Woman was Jessica Davis. Yes, I just blew her cover. She's stunningly beautiful and makes the perfect tall, strong, gorgeous, and curvy Wonder Woman. She fits the part to a T and is crazy sweet to everyone she meets. She's become a great friend, and our whole team thinks the world of her. As runners passed Wonder Woman and me at the start line, they waved, cheered, shouted, and stopped for selfies. They did the same thing on their way through the finish. Sometimes it's almost unfair to call my profession "work."

Beth Salinger is an experienced, strong, and thoughtful leader who always prioritizes her crew. My stage for the start and finish line was

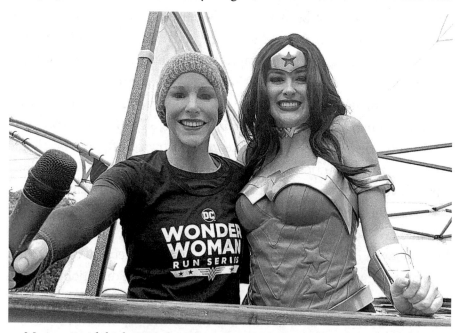

My iconic sidekick, Wonder Woman. Jay Sutherland/Sport Photo Group

a little unusual, so she got creative to keep me warm and dry. I was working from a 1-person contraption that resembled the tall structure a drum major would stand on while conducting a marching band. Since the stage wasn't a typical stage, it couldn't support the typical canopy used to protect me and the high-tech equipment. But Beth wouldn't be deterred. Instead, she asked our team to build a chain link fence around my stage, and then affixed a canopy to that.

They also gave me a space heater, which sat at my feet and kept me toasty throughout the morning. It was another fine example of individuals going all out to help me through this nightmare.

Race morning was a huge success. And, even though I didn't get to see more than my hotel and the start line in Little Rock, I left appreciating that the people there were total gamers. At 3 p.m., I boarded another plane, which would get me to Atlanta and then Detroit by 10 p.m. I was about 85% of the way through conquering my big 3-state tour. I was drained, but also eager to see my Goddesses in the morning for our annual love fest on Mother's Day. When I arrived at my hotel, my sweet friends and members of my online training group The Hottie Body Fitness Challenge, Jason and Katie Stefaniak, welcomed me with a humidifier. They are two of the most diehard members of the group I lovingly refer to as my Hotties. My Stefaniaks are wonderful people, and I'm proud of all they've accomplished using my Exact Formula for Weight Loss. And because I had chosen not to speak once I left Little Rock, I was hoping I'd still have my voice in the morning.

May 12. Sunday.

Delighted to have woken up with a voice, I jumped in the car with the Stefaniaks and headed to the Ann Arbor Goddess races. I can't say enough nice things about this race director, Eva Solomon. We met in 2014 when I was working for another company and have become very good friends since then. She introduced herself to the group as a race director and then I introduced myself as an announcer. I've been hosting her Goddess-themed races every year since. She puts on about 17 high-quality endurance events annually, and I'm happy to add some spunk, energy, and love to those I announce.

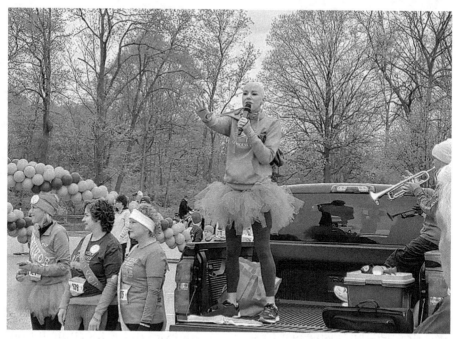

With a few ovarian cancer survivors at the Ann Arbor Goddess 5k.
Photo by Greg Sadler

One of the things I like best about Eva (on a very long list), is that she's downright confident with who she is and not remotely catty to other women. She's a legit athlete who's completed IRONMAN™ triathlons, marathons, and more. She's a rockstar business owner who manages a strong team with a confident, but easy approach. I mention her lack of cattiness because, sadly, there's still a lot of that floating around. I'm of the attitude that we can all win, and I'm excited to work with excellent people of any gender. And so is Eva. I cringe when I come across a few of the gals in the running industry who are very mean-spirited behind closed doors. Women who outwardly claim to support women and then do the opposite behind their backs. I've been the target of it. It's fine because I'm sturdy and thriving despite their efforts. Still, it's disheartening to see. Eva is the real deal though. Her company, Epic Races, employs a diverse crew and her Goddess races really do provide an awesome environment for all. She's also gorgeous and has amazing muscles. That's a sidebar, though!

The Ann Arbor Goddess races are something I always look forward to, but that I also fear. I'll explain. The event hosts about 1,000 people annually and it partners with the Michigan Ovarian Cancer Alliance. While 1,000 is a solid group of people, it's small enough to be very personal. We always have a few dozen ovarian cancer survivors and patients participate, and sometimes it scares the bejeezus out of me. Eva provides our survivors and patients with teal sashes, which makes them easily identifiable. Ever since my first year, I've gone out of my way to meet them individually and bestow immense amounts of love as they start and as they finish their race. I greet them with hugs, praise them by name, and generally raise a stink. During my first year announcing it, I met a standout participant, Heather Cook Gilbeau. She was a young mom who had been diagnosed in January, four months prior. She showed up with a buzz cut from chemo, a teal tutu, and a smile. I was in complete awe of Heather and quickly got to know her story while doing my thing. We instantly became friends on Facebook and shared a few sweet messages. But within a few months, she passed away. That really really hurt. Ovarian cancer is scary. Yes, breast cancer is, too. But I think ovarian cancer is a bit more intimidating because it's difficult to detect in the early stages. It doesn't have as high of a cure rate. In addition to Heather, these races had led me to meet and fall quickly in love with a ton of other women. Fun, athletic, vibrant women of all ages whom I will always dread losing. Every year when I go back, I have a little list in my head of goddesses that I need to check off the list as "alive." I honestly care about them so much. How that happens from these quick, annual interactions, I don't know. But it does.

Erica Jo Earle was another heartbreaker. This 30-something participated in the 2017 one-miler. She was pushed in a wheelchair by a huge pack of family members and friends who came out to support her. They were all wearing white Team Erica shirts, and they were so somber. All of them. Erica was visibly very sick. She was pale, frail, and bald with big beautiful blue eyes. Her head hung low, and it was apparent that she felt like hell. I gave the appropriate shout outs for Team Erica at the start line and joined the group as they approached the finish line. Like I did with all of the other beautiful sash-wearing women, I bent down and gave Erica a big hug. I told her something like "We all love you and are so happy you're here." Poor thing was listless. It was a wonderful showing of love and support, but it was agonizingly painful for everyone involved. I hated the thought of this lovely young woman losing her life and how sad that would make everyone who loved her. As they crossed their finish line, I hung back trying to mask my tears. I left Michigan with a dagger stuck in my heart. Erica passed away about five months later. These moments and these people will stay in my heart forever.

As I pulled up to the event with the Stefaniaks, I took a deep breath and hoped to see all of my friends. Usually, Eva has a teal tutu made for me, but this year, she gave me a pink tutu and a teal hoodie instead. Even though I hate being anything other than a supporter of those on the course, I think my friends in Ann Arbor felt a bit of solidarity with me. They've always known how much I adore them, but this time, they all let me know how much they cared for me. Cancer is the thing nobody wants to have in common, but there we were, pink tutus and teal tutus standing together. We all knew the traumas associated with the big C,

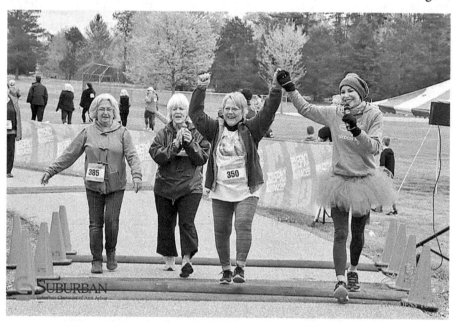

Crossing with Erica's mom, Joanne. Photo by Greg Sadler.

which made the hugs pretty real. My job was still to fawn all over these beautiful ladies, entertain the masses, and make sure everyone in the crowd knew how vital healthy habits, annual screenings, and funding was. So, I took to my pre-race stage, which was the back of a pickup truck, brought over as many survivors as possible to join me, took off my hat, and made my case. Once again, my bald head worked its magic in quieting the crowd. Many of the participants would later tell me that they experienced chills and that they would take cancer prevention and detection more seriously. After that, my sole intention for the day was to deliver big fun!

Once I yelled "GO" I spent the next two hours dancing, hugging, and warmly welcoming all of my athletes, especially those beautiful gals in teal blue sashes, to and through the finish line. I greeted them each like they'd just earned Olympic gold, and they returned the love ten-fold. We had so much fun laughing, dancing, and cruising hand-in-hand through the finish. It was a wonderful day for everyone involved. Erica Jo Earle's mom Joanne Erickson had returned for the third year in a row. We met when Team Erica returned in 2018, and it was a real treat to see smiles on their faces. They were our final finishers that year, and as they approached the finish line, someone alerted me to the fact that Joanne was Erica's mom. I greeted her with the biggest hug, and she squeezed me back tightly. I stayed put and asked everyone to celebrate Erica, as Joanne and her crew threw their arms up in the air. It took me a bit to compose myself once again.

Back to 2019, I felt a bit guilty about showing up with cancer because I didn't want Joanne to have to worry. When she arrived, we shared a lengthy embrace and I assured her that I was going to be okay. This time, we held hands as she crossed the finish line and boldly celebrated the life of her beautiful daughter. In my book, nothing in the world could be worse than losing a child. It meant so much to me to see Joanne happy and to be able to enjoy this Mother's Day.

Another highlight for me was the turnout of my Hotties. Michigan is full of them and they swarm to any event I announce. Post-race, about a dozen of us went to Zingerman's, the famous local deli, to catch up, talk about fitness, and share some laughs. Everyone had something new and exciting to discuss. How I've lucked out with so many wonderful people in my life, I have no idea.

When I headed to the airport that afternoon, I was physically whooped, but still felt incredibly triumphant. This was one hell of a 10-day gauntlet, and I conquered every freaking one of my challenges. I definitely had a scare with my voice, but I earned it back in the nick of time and was able to give my races and athletes the massive doses of noisy love they deserved. I know I didn't beat anyone, but I definitely felt like I had won something. Point awarded to … Fitz Koehler!

The following week was monopolized by rest and tedious doctor appointments. I also got to do some special momming. Parker had his 8th-grade prom and he looked extra sharp in the outfit he and Rob had bought. It was a stylish outfit with gray slacks and a light blue long-sleeved button-down shirt. Black tie, shoes, and belt. Swoon! I scored a sweet pre-dance pic with him kissing my cheek, and that fixed everything for the moment. I was so happy not to miss any of their special occasions.

Despite the special moments with my Beans, life was really rough. When I wasn't with them, I was breaking down, and crying nonstop. The constant stomach explosions were horrible to live with, as were the other side effects. At some point, one of my fingernails got caught in a drawer, pulled up a little bit, and I squealed with pain. I thought that it was a weird one-off deal, but it wasn't. Since fingernails and toenails consist of quickly replicating cells, mine were being destroyed by chemo. The constant pain of catching my nails on anything and everything caused me to file them extra short. But, no matter how short I went, they were continuously pulling up and ripping off. The parts of my nails that remained were turning yellow and developing strange ridges. I hadn't been warned about this. Every round of chemo led to a new ridge and a new cycle of nail death. Do you know how the rings of a tree trunk represent the tree's age? Each yellow, rainbow-shaped ridge on my nails represented a round of chemo. It was bizarre. It felt like any time I touched anything, I was yelping. I tried to cover all of my fingertips with bandages, but it was a futile effort. The fun continued when my toenails started ripping off, too. My ogre-look was becoming complete. To make things even more fun, my hands were becoming incredibly weak— I couldn't open jars, cans, or boxes. Life was growing more complicated and difficult, and I was careening toward Chemo #4.

May 20. Monday.

Round #4. Going back in for chemo was crazy stressful. The process wasn't the problem, but knowing what it was going to do to me was. While everyone in the world thought I was brave, I was actually sobbing on my way to the cancer center. I couldn't even talk to Rob about it. I'd just sit there and nervously cry. But, even with that fear and stress on my chest, I got out of the car and put one foot in front of the other until I was sitting in that recliner, having a needle poked into my chest. Lilly was on a trip to Europe for this round, so I saw nurse John Colon instead. I used to be his mom's personal trainer and have been friends with the entire family since. John was the perfect replacement for Lilly. He had a great disposition, and was super funny, sarcastic, and precise. I'd seen him a few times for IV fluids before, so I had no surprises. Once my port was accessed, John drew some blood to send back to the lab for testing. One of Dr. Gordan's nurses, Holli Carvajal, APRN, came out to tell me that while I was given permission to have chemo, they were concerned about my hemoglobin (HGB) counts. That was a conversation Dr. Gordan had been having with me for a while. My HGB counts kept dropping lower and lower each week, and he didn't like it. My question was always, "What can I do to combat this proactively?" The answer was always "nothing." Helpless to fix myself, I sat down for my cocktail of Benadryl, steroids, and chemo drugs.

In an effort to keep my family happy, I agreed to go see *End Game,* Marvel's newest superhero movie, after a long nap. It had been out for almost a month already, and everyone had waited patiently for me to be in town and free to see it. While I was concerned about falling asleep halfway through, we've loved all of the Marvel movies, and I particularly love Thor, so they really didn't have to twist my arm to get me to go.

About halfway through the movie, I heard a strange musical beeping sound. At first, I thought it was part of the movie, but as I turned around to see where it was coming from, I saw a child sitting on a woman's lap playing a video game. The volume was on high and I instantly blurted out, "Turn that thing off!" Then I turned back toward the movie screen and waited. Thirty seconds went by. Sixty seconds went by, and that music was still blaring. So, once again, I whipped my head around and scolded "Turn that thing off, NOW!" At this point, I was boiling up inside and planning to give her about 10 more seconds before I climbed over my chair, ripped that thing out of the kid's hand, and tossed it in the trash. There was zero consideration for walking around the aisles of chairs to get to them. I was literally on the brink of hurdling my chair when thankfully, the music stopped playing. The kid started crying, and his dad carried him out. I'm considering this great fortune for all of us involved. Apparently, the steroids from that morning were running hot through my blood, and I could have ended up on national news. I can just imagine the headlines. "Fitz Smash! Crazy Bald Woman Starts Benching-Clearing Brawl During *End Game* in a Case of Roid Rage." That or the usual "Florida Woman" in a really funny story that'd make my entire state look bad.

May 22. Wednesday.

While most sane people in my position were resting, I was preparing to host my annual Morning Mile skating party. That's where I invite all Morning Milers in Alachua County to attend, which is about 20 schools worth of people. It's a free party I host every year where we celebrate every step taken and acknowledge major accomplishments, such as kids who've completed more than 100 miles, with special rewards. Usually between 800 -1,000 people attend. Despite my sickness, I was eager to see all of my kids. My mom and big brother John were also headed into town for a visit. It was the first time I'd seen John since my diagnosis and I couldn't wait to spend time with him. He's an incredible human being: Smart, caring, thoughtful, successful, handsome, easy-going, and really funny. We have a bunch of things in common, including our love of sports, sunshine, and Jeep Wranglers. We were also both BALD! I couldn't wait to get a picture of us with matching heads, and it was one of the first things we did when they arrived. We took shots head-on, side profiles, and pics with our tongues out. They're hysterical. My mom always thought we kind of looked alike, but once we stood side by side without my long hair to distract, the similarity was uncanny.

I took my entire family to the skating rink with me for the event, and they were happy to go. I spent a couple of hours greeting and congratulating countless Morning Milers, their families, and the teachers involved. I took the microphone to announce the award ceremony, passed out a multitude of rewards, and basked in the success of my program. As usual, everything went smoothly. I'm lucky to have had the best backup plan in the world that evening though. If I was too sick to attend, Ginger was going to fill in for me. She knows my program like the back of her hand, has attended the previous eight skating parties, and is a total rock star on the microphone. Poised, confident, and well-spoken. When the party was over, my family headed to a Japanese steakhouse for dinner.

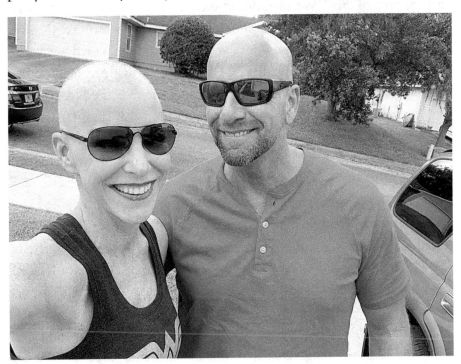

Twinning with my big brother, John.

While I didn't eat much, I was satisfied simply being able to spend time with the people that I loved. Rob had been taking first-class care of me, but it would have been really nice to have my mom and John visit more often.

May 24. Friday

Rob hugged me, sighed, and shook his head as I headed toward TSA. Severe chemo sickness had kicked in at its worst and I was struggling. Boarding a plane four days after chemo #4 to go host my most demanding marathon weekend of the year was close to insane. But if I had to do it again, I'd choose insanity over surrender every time. My destination was The Buffalo Marathon, which takes place on Memorial Day Weekend and, like me, oozes total patriotism. Everything is decked out in red, white, and blue, the people are highly motivated, and the variety of races keeps things moving. Lastly, I love the race's director, Greg Weber, who has become a very close friend. I met Greg at a running conference in February of 2017. We introduced ourselves one afternoon and I remember him asking me, "Why should we hire you for our event?" Greg was using a local DJ at that point, which nobody was blown away by. I told him that while he busted his butt all year creating the event, on race day everyone thinks the person on the microphone is the race director. Did he want Pee Wee Herman or Mick Jagger in that role? He thought about it, laughed, and asked if I was free Memorial Day weekend. He then asked who else I announced for. I responded with my usual list, including Big Sur Marathon, Los Angeles Marathon, and the OC Marathon. Greg asked me to pencil his race into my calendar, I agreed, and we parted ways. He then made a beeline for Big Sur's Doug Thurston and asked what he thought about me. Doug replied with some derivative of, "Book her now!" and Greg boomeranged back and told me to lock his date in with Sharpie. The exchange describes Greg to a T. He's smart, open-minded, well-researched, and quick to make decisions that benefit his race. He takes amazing care of me every year and we always do something fun like visit Niagara Falls or hike in the scenic gorges nearby. The rest of the year, we stay in touch weekly. His friendship is one of the very special things I would have truly missed out on, if not for my role in the running community.

Poor Greg was also the victim of my request for IV fluids during race weekend. I felt bad asking, but this was the support I needed. He had a million race details to manage and booking hydration for his announcer was piled on top as another thing to do. Unsurprisingly, Greg and our Buffalo Marathon Medical Director made it happen. My flight arrived at noon and I was scheduled to be picked up from the airport by Greg and Dave McGillvray who is the race director for the Boston Marathon. Dave's another good guy. Via text, I was told to take the exit by baggage claim and wait for them in the parking garage across the way. I did what I was told and stood in that freezing garage for about 10 minutes until finally, I called Greg and was given the "Oops! Sorry. Not the garage. We're parked on the road outside of baggage pickup." Okay. So, back I went. Greg and Dave were working on their phones as I walked up, barely acknowledging me. They gave me awkward hugs and then basically stood there watching as I was about to load my bags into the back of the SUV. Umm. Okay. I was totally confused at this point because I was pretty sure they both knew I was all about manners and chivalry and, technically, so were they. And it was extra bizarre because I was also their cancer patient lady friend. Why wouldn't they help me with my luggage? I decided that manners must not have been their thing at the moment, so I started to pick up my big bag to load it up. Just then, out popped one very noisy man. It was Rudy! Surprise! Greg invited him to come to Buffalo and work with me in case I needed help. Rudy and I had a big hug, Greg caught it on video, and happiness was had. Truth be told, I had been encouraging Greg to bring Rudy to Buffalo for years. Greg always said that I was all he needed, but I knew once he experienced us as a team, he'd always want Rudy to return as well.

We drove straight to the Hyatt hotel where a nurse from Revive: Buffalo's Hydration Station was waiting for me. Greg had also provided me with a tray full of apple juice bottles, since at the time, besides water, it was the only thing I could drink. This was a pretty awesome experience because I got to put on the cozy hotel bathrobe (I'm obsessed with cozy

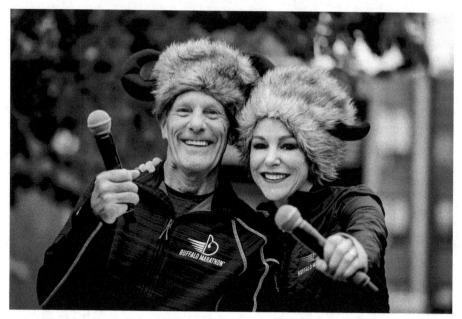

My Junior Poobah and me, the Grand Poobah! Photo by Jeff Tracy

bathrobes), lie down in bed, watch TV, and chill out while the saline dripped into my arm. It would have been luxurious if all of my infusions were given to me this way. After about an hour, the nurse was gone and I was able to rest up for that night's VIP party. Once again, I chose to fake feeling good and did my best to look fabulous. I threw on my red wrap dress and showed up with a smile on my face. Socializing was a little tiring, but time with my Buffalo friends was definitely worth the effort. In the past I'd go out with the team to a sports bar afterward, but not this year. My bed was calling my name and I needed major rest.

May 25. Saturday.

We kicked the morning off with the Buffalo Marathon 5K and 2,000 excited runners, including Rudy, taking to the downtown streets. Since I have run so many of Rudy's races over time, it's an awesome opportunity to get to welcome him across a finish line. He's a very experienced runner with a couple of sub-three-hour marathons in his past. Our athletes were in great spirits, despite some rain, while I enjoyed being dry announcing from underneath a lovely canopy. Rudy won second place in his age group and then joined me on the mic not too long after he crossed the finish line.

Next up was the Diaper Dash! Yes, please. I could have done this all day. Inside the Buffalo Convention Center, our team laid out a beautiful custom-made Diaper Dash floor mat so that cuties ages two and under could conquer 26.2 feet. I would greet about 10 of them at a time and then yell "Baby Buffaloes, GO!" Then, those adorable babies would crawl, roll, drool, or toddle toward the other end of the mat. Others would roam around in circles or sit and cry. No matter what, the amount of excitement the parents and grandparents exuded was massive. Clearly, those baby buffaloes could do no wrong. The star of the show was Greg's newborn granddaughter, Maci, whom I'm pretty sure he had in mind when he created the dash. While announcing to these beautiful, bald little people, I was beginning to learn that associating with other baldies was a good idea.

The Kids Mini Marathon for ages three to eight brought us back on the street leading up to our grand finish line. I loved being down on the road with these families. They were bursting with energy and brought boundless joy to racing. As a big-picture fitness pro, I adore seeing the pride parents have while pursuing fitness with their children. I always tell them, "You think you're just out for a fun Saturday morning with your kids. However, you are also setting the stage for them to pursue a lifetime of athletic adventure and the healthy habits that go along with it. This stuff matters!" I enjoy seeing that resonate with the parents. My hope is that they'll continue to make sports and fitness a dominant component of their family's culture. Once I gave some quick safety instructions, hosted a daddy dance party, and reminded the kids to smile big at the finish line with their hands up high, I yelled "GO" a bunch of times for a bunch of little waves. Everything that happened between our start and the finish line was pure magic. Lots of proud speedsters, confused slower runners and, inevitably, a few criers. A handful of kids took a tumble and bounced back up. A few of our less confident tots needed someone to hold their hand, and guess who was more than happy to do that? Me! In Buffalo, we have a few kids who just make our hearts explode. Often, with an inspiring non-profit organization called Footsteps of Western New York. Some of them include superstars with cerebral palsy and spina bifida who take to the streets with their braces and walkers. Being a part of an inclusive event where all children have an equal opportunity to perform and earn their reward is more than special. Time with our challenged athletes rips my heart out and heals it all at the same time. To heck with cancer! These kids were legit warriors and I had nothing to complain about.

Richard Clark is the other Buffalo Marathon Race Director. While Greg manages the business side of things, Rich takes care of operations. They are a dynamic duo who complement each other like peas and carrots. Rich is a schoolteacher who also loves starting the longer distance races for the older kids. Between Rich, Rudy, and myself, every child received a mega-dose of instruction and enthusiasm. These races are so adorable and entertaining that even people without kids stick around to watch. They're as much of a spectator sport as anything else. Our next event was, too.

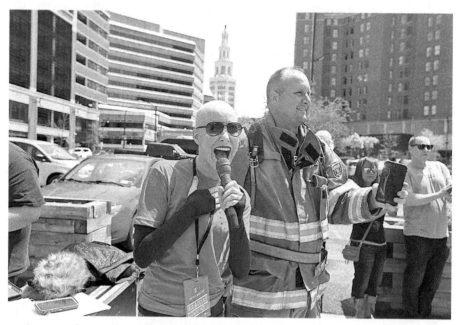

Singing the anthem, with firefighter Ryan Mast. Photo by James McCoy

This was the second running of The Ruffalo Stampede, a 1K race for K-9s and their human companions. It's quickly become a highlight of the entire weekend. One of the most notable things about the 200+ dogs gathered together is how well-behaved and kind they all were. Seriously. There was no biting, growling, or snarling at all. My philosophy on that is that if a person cares enough about their dog to take it to a doggie race, that person likely has also invested time and energy into raising it properly. Our selection of good dogs included everything from saint bernards and chihuahuas, to poodles, and pitbulls. Rudy manned the finish line, and I conducted the start while playing dog-themed music. Our athletes got to know each other with plenty of tail wagging, booty sniffing, and happy barking.

A few minutes before it was time to yell "GO," I quieted the crowd for the national anthem, as sung by LeAnn Rimes via my iPad. As the crowd hushed and stood at attention, I pressed play and LeAnn belted out, "Oh, say can you see" and then … NOTHING. The music stopped and I quickly looked at my iPad to figure out what went wrong. Since it had been sitting out in the sun, it had overheated and died. Ugh. Perfect freaking timing. So I had to do something that would bring great harm to the ears of everyone. I brought the microphone to my mouth and started singing, "by the dawn's early light …" Since my voice is not good at all, I sang into the microphone held in my right hand and used the left hand to encourage the crowd to sing with me. Thankfully they complied and I was able to turn my horrible solo into a beautiful patriotic sing-along. Even the doggies howled. Yikes. I might be an atrocious singer, but I love America more than I love my ego. I was not going to let the anthem just die there on that street. If you ever need a laugh, just envision me and my bald head, singing off-key to a big group in Buffalo with the dogs howling in response.

After launching the Stampede, I hustled over to the finish line to meet Rudy. We had a blast welcoming our spirited athletes and their owners, which dragged behind them on leashes. Once the last pup earned its finishers tag for its collar, I went straight to the Hyatt for more IV fluids.

May 26. Sunday.

I was so happy to walk with Rudy toward the start line for the Buffalo Marathon and Half Marathon. It wasn't that I needed help announcing, but more like races are just more fun when we're together. It's no secret that Rudy has been doing this way longer than I have, but I've caught up pretty quickly and we stand as equals on stages. Well, that's usually the case. But in Buffalo, he was the new guy at *my* race. As you can imagine, I took the opportunity to torture him. Since I announce the races wearing a big horned Buffalo hat, which kind of resembles Fred Flintstone's "Grand Poobah" hat, many people call me the Grand Poobah of the Buffalo Marathon. Clearly that would make Rudy the "Junior Poobah", so I called him that publicly all weekend. I had brought a second, shorter Buffalo hat to add variety to my attire, but since Rudy showed up without warning, I made him wear it instead. He did so graciously and the runners got a kick out of it. The mood was electric as more than 5,000 athletes formed the largest herd of "buffalo" in the United States at that moment. Once I yelled "GO" the stampede began and we enjoyed the thunderous roar of runners as they passed our stage hooting, hollering, and kicking up their heels.

The morning was cold and very windy. I kept busy dancing on our stage and running around the finish line chute with our athletes just to keep warm. Anything to help fend off my shivers. We had a bunch of personal friends out on the course and kept track of them using the Buffalo Marathon app. When one of them approached, I would run down to give congratulatory hugs and escort them through the finish line. In a nutshell, my day was hella active. Not something you'd expect from a girl who'd had a vicious dose of chemo at the beginning of her week, but totally believable for a person who loves athletes and was totally juiced up on adrenaline. Like with the OC Marathon, I was somewhat asking for trouble.

As Captain Obvious would have predicted, Greg loved the way we operated together and said that he would definitely invite Rudy back the next year. Score! We welcomed our final finisher around 3 p.m. and I was toast. I wasn't just tired, I was the kind of tired that made me think something was really wrong. But since I was used to feeling horrible and didn't want to alarm anyone, I remained on autopilot and kept quiet. Greg hosted a dinner for a group of us later that night, but the whole thing was a blur. I couldn't really eat anything and simple conversation hurt my throat and my head. My body had definitely hit a new low. I bowed out early and returned to the Hyatt to crash.

May 27. Monday.

Happy birthday to me. Oy. While I was appreciative of being able to grow another year older, I wasn't necessarily in the physical or mental shape to celebrate. I had to fly home that afternoon and the thought of going to the airport made me cry. For real. After a wonderful weekend, in which I wouldn't have changed any of my efforts, every move I made burdened my poor body. My levels of sickness and fatigue were extreme and I wasn't sure how to go about fixing them. Greg drove me to the airport and I landed back in Gainesville to my sweet family by 5:30 p.m.

Rob, Ginger, and Parker picked me up, excited to take me out for a birthday dinner. Honestly, the last thing I wanted to do was go anywhere other than my bed, but I wanted to give them the opportunity to celebrate, so off to Piesano's we went. My treatments hadn't made their lives easy and they deserved a decent night out. Remaining upright through dinner was hard, but I was happy to be with them. When we returned home, they brought out my cake and sang Happy Birthday. Cookie dough ice cream cake coated with Magic Shell and chocolate-covered strawberries has been my go-to for many years. And while I couldn't really stomach it, I enjoyed that they got it for me and that we could spend time together. I also really enjoyed passing out shortly after.

May 28. Tuesday.

I didn't feel any better as I headed in for IV fluids with Rob, who took the day off work because I looked far worse than usual. I had become accustomed to feeling terrible, but once again, I had discovered a new low. When we arrived at the cancer center, several of the nurses were startled to see me so sickly and gray and I was quickly shuttled to a chair in the back of the room for an evaluation. My blood was drawn and when the results returned, they delivered bad news. My hemoglobin numbers had plummeted too far, and I needed blood transfusions. The thought of some strangers' blood being imported into my body grossed me out beyond belief. No way. No how. Yuck! But the medical team explained how thoroughly donated blood was screened and cleaned (especially for immunocompromised cancer patients) and exactly how much I needed it. If I didn't accept two bags of blood now, I'd require even more of it later. This was a nightmare, and worse yet, we had to go next door to the actual hospital to get those grody bags of stranger blood. I had no interest in going to the hospital for anything, but those were the rules, so off we went. It took about an hour to get checked in, but one of the worst blows came when I realized what was REALLY going on. I thought I was just going to be sitting in some sort of mini infusion room getting the transfusions for a couple of hours before I went home. Wrong! I was being brought into my own room on the oncology floor to be admitted overnight. The second I stepped into that room and saw the bed with the gown on top of it, I started sobbing. I was devastated. If you remember, not being hospitalized was first on my list of mini-goals. It was symbolic of me being in a bad place health-wise and it completely broke my heart. Obviously, this all coincided with how badly I felt. I clearly needed medical attention, but I despised all of it. I was sick of being mortal.

The first nurse that was assigned to me was youngish, sweet, and caring. I appreciated her kindness, but she was lacking some important skills. She tried to access my port and screwed that up by using a needle that was too short. So, the needle went through my chest, but wasn't long enough to make it through the actual port. As a reminder, having a needle poked into that spot hurt like a mother. She wanted to try again with a longer needle, but I refused. That was a one-shot deal. I told her she could use my arm, but after digging another needle around in there for a while, she failed at that too. Then I told her she was no longer allowed to poke me with anything, anywhere, ever again. It's amazing how many medical professionals have "oohed and ahhed" over my veins in the past. I'm lean and kind of vascular and they usually think I'm an easy stick. I am not. Not at all. In fact, everyone on the planet other than Lilly and John usually screw it up.

Once I refused access to nurse #1, I explained to the head nurse lady that if they wanted to stick me again, they were going to have to get their absolute finest, most experienced nurse to do it. And if that person screwed it up, I would be going home. Unfortunately for me, that experienced person was Nurse Ratched. Man, she was one unpleasant soul and she ended up being assigned to me for the entire night. I needed someone with top-notch skills, but I also really needed some sweetness and compassion. I got neither. While I knew bags of yuck were going to be dripping into me, I didn't want to see them and I

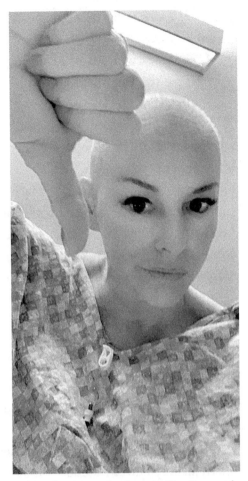

Thumbs down for hospitalization and stranger blood.

requested that my IV pole be placed behind my line of vision. Nurse Ratched didn't care. She never smiled or showed concern. She never asked how I felt or if I needed anything. She just stomped around with a cranky face leaving big gross bags of "stranger blood" in plain view. She also left some nasty gauze pads soaked with my own blood at the foot of the bed overnight, something I didn't notice until the following morning. Not okay. Just two days prior, I was the Grand Poobah running the streets of Buffalo with thousands of athletes. How the hell did I go from that to this? And poor Rob. He spent the night at the hospital concerned because:

1. His sick wife was being poked in all of the wrong ways and made to cry.
2. His sick wife was threatening to walk out of the hospital and refuse the treatment she desperately needed because of incompetence.

It wasn't an awesome night, but I got through it. I was still exhausted when I woke up, but the transfusion process was over. I kept trying to imagine what the people that were now flowing through my veins were like. I couldn't conjure up any physical traits, but I did decide that they simply must have been nice people. Blood donors are pretty great, right? I was shocked that I was now a blood recipient. It was another rude welcome into The Twilight Zone. Fortunately, Nurse Ratched took her miserable self home before 7 a.m. I was happy she was gone.

Before I was able to check out and leave this hell, the head nurse came into my room to see how my night was. While nothing I said was going to undo the bad experiences I had, I spoke up for the folks that would soon be lying in my bed. This was the oncology floor. While I was youngish and healthy-ish and had a great caregiver, many of the people checking in were old, frail, and alone. I could only imagine how many people had died in the room I spent the night in. It saddened me to think that anyone would spend their last day or night on earth being mistreated by Nurse Ratched. I told the head nurse about my awful care and explained how I was treated like an inanimate object. I felt as if I was just a car having my tire changed, instead of feeling like a person being gently cared for. She seemed to take that analogy to heart and asked if she could share it at her team meeting. Hopefully that conversation helped the next person. I've always felt fortunate not to be surrounded by my generational peers at the cancer center. I rarely see people my age, which is a great thing. But, it's really hard to see so many elderly people, often dropped off by some sort of van driver, left alone in the lobby until they're retrieved. It's even worse when after their treatments they're left in a wheelchair to wait for the van driver who may or may not come quickly. Even on my hardest days, I wanted to take some of the older folks home and care for them. They often appeared so helpless. I definitely believed that everyone was getting elite medical care from the team at FCS, but I also wanted them to be surrounded by a loving family. That's another reason why I could never have a pity party for myself. There was always someone who had it worse.

I decided not to tell anyone about my hospital stay, with the exception of a handful of close friends and family. I can only imagine the fallout if I had shared some pathetic picture of me on social media. No, thank you! While I'm certain the kindness would have overflowed from my phone, that's not the type of attention I wanted. I was clear from the get-go. I did not want pity, which a sickly picture post from the hospital would have certainly garnered. I'd been sharing a little from chemo or doctor's appointments, but I kept those posts light. I often used silly Snapchat filters when doing so. I was allowing the public in on my experience in a bright and airy way without ever discussing the actual hardships. My cancer treatment, my choice. I just wanted to keep this train moving without a bunch of panic or sadness. It's funny how many people would reach out to say, "You're doing so great!" or "You look so healthy!" In reality, neither of those things were true. I was sick as a dog and underneath my foundation and lipstick, I was a hot mess. But everyone was thinking exactly what I wanted them to think. My family and I would often joke that my Academy Award was on its way.

Fitzness Log

Chemo #3 destroyed me. When I wasn't at FCS to get chemo or IV fluids, all I was capable of doing was sleep. My muscles were completely depleted of energy, and I can confidently count this as the first month of my life since I was a toddler that I didn't do some sort of deliberate exercise. While I'm obviously a strong proponent of being active, doing so at this point would have been detrimental.

Chapter 6

When Things Go Wrong, Don't Go With Them (Naked in the Airport)

June 7. Friday.

Parker and I boarded our plane to Chicago, Illinois for the DC Wonder Woman Run Series. It was tradition to fly my kids with me for one work trip every year, and this was his turn. He's an incredibly wise and insightful kid, but sometimes he's only talkative when he's fully relaxed and away from daily burdens like school, chores, and sports. His biting wit can cause me to explode with laughter in an instant, so sharing some quality alone time with Mr. Parker was something I had looked forward to for a long time. My race directors had generously booked us a room at the Great Wolf Lodge and I was praying I would feel healthy enough to fully enjoy it with him. If you're unfamiliar, it's a family-friendly resort with a large indoor water park and an array of fun activities, such as bowling, rock wall climbing, mini-golf, and more. When we arrived, we were given wolf ear headbands, which we proudly wore as much as possible. We checked into our cute little log cabin themed room where Parker had his own little space with bunk beds.

We tossed on our swimsuits and headed straight for the water park. Although we only stayed for about an hour, we rode quite a few slides and splashed around in the lazy river. Climbing up the stairs to get to the slides was pretty taxing, but I tried to suck it up so Parker wouldn't be burdened or notice I was feeling unwell. My focus was on making sure he had some genuine fun and I think we both did.

In fact, I think the entire weekend was a hit. My sister-in-law, Sandy, and nephew, Johnny, were in town, so we dined with them a couple of times and the trio ran the 5K together. They all lined up together, but Parker and Sandy finished the race ahead of Johnny. That turned out to be a win for me because I got to run through the finish line, hand-in-hand, with my sweet nephew.

When we had some leisure time at the resort, Parker and I explored the extensive amenities and made good use of *almost* all of them. We absolutely dominated the mini-bowling alley, competed against each other in world-championship-worthy air hockey battles, and faced our fears completing the above-ground ropes course. We also broke my traditional healthy mom rules and bought appalling amounts of candy, which made him very happy. It seems that, like with my athletes, I was able to ignore sick feelings for my children too. Point awarded to … Fitz and Parker Koehler!

We threw some new stuff into our DC Wonder Woman Run Series races this weekend. Our 5,000 athletes got to run through the Six Flags Theme Park, which is loaded up with tons of themed rides and displays dedicated to DC Comics. It was a cohesive pairing for our run series and our athletes gushed about the experience. The energy at our start lines was sublime and I particularly enjoyed that my nephew, Johnny, had so much fun. He had never run an organized race before and it tickled me to see his happy face beaming from the middle of the crowd as I led the start line shenanigans. He is 6'3", so even though he was behind at least 2,000 other people, it was easy for me to see his ginormous smile from the stage. I wanted him to have a quality experience, so it meant a lot to me to see him happy. Who knows? If he didn't have fun, he may never want to participate in a race again! Instead, he declared that he loved every minute of it. And hearing, "Aunt Fitz, you are really good at race announcing," didn't hurt either.

I had a ton of friends come out to see me in Chicago, which made my heart really happy. I was told that 200 people used my discount code "Fitzness" when they registered and I'm pretty sure that I actually knew them all. This is especially neat because I've never announced a race anywhere in the entire state of Illinois before.

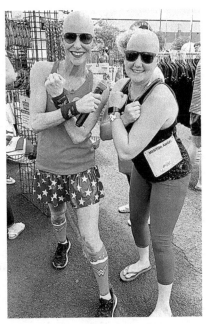

Proud to twin with my runners fighting cancer!

I am constantly amazed by how many friends I've amassed around the USA and beyond thanks to my career. I've lived in Florida my entire life, which makes having a bunch of buddies in the other 49 states pretty cool. Our runners and walkers love to race, travel, and meet people; being on the receiving end of so much goodness often makes me pinch myself.

I also spent time with a new friend who drove about two hours into town just to have me autograph some photos he'd printed out. I laughed when he apologized because the photos were of me with hair. All I could think was, "Hey bud. That's still me! I may look different now, but those old pics still count." Truth be told, I personally preferred photos of me with my hair, so I didn't mind at all. And speaking of not having hair, I met two beautiful bald athletes who were also going through chemo. One had breast cancer and one had leukemia; both were really lovely, and I envied their ability to race. This is the perfect example of every cancer diagnosis, treatment, and response being as unique as a fingerprint. While I wasn't up for exercise, I was genuinely happy that they were. We laughed a bit about our bald heads, discussed our treatment plans, and took a few pics. From start to finish, our participants rocked their Wonder Woman gear and celebrated with every step they took. I did my best to bring big joy from the microphone, and they returned the favor with endless smiles all weekend. Despite all of the Wonder Women and superheroes who won the day, my fondest memories of Chicago came from the quality time I'd spent with Parker Beans. As soon as we flew home, I was headed straight back to chemo.

June 12. Wednesday.

It was time for chemo #5 And I was pretty beat up. My ability to bounce back was getting worse and it was stressful to watch myself continuously deteriorate without any ability to fully recover. Adrenaline still fueled me for race announcing, but every other moment was filled with exhaustion, evil stomach explosions, and some sort of pain from my nails ripping off, black and blue triceps, sore quads, etc. When I started chemo, people would say that the side effects were cumulative. I didn't really understand what they meant back then, but recently I've decided that it's kind of like a boxing match (kickboxing for me). The first few times you get hit aren't too bad. But as the 5th, 8th, and 10th rounds arrive, each strike lands harder than the last. This happens even if the strikes aren't any more powerful. Why? Well, the first kick in the ribs feels bad and does a small bit of damage. But when your opponent keeps kicking you in the same place, round after round, those later kicks become excruciating. Do you remember a blood-soaked Rocky at the end of his movie battles shouting, "Is that all you've got?" Of

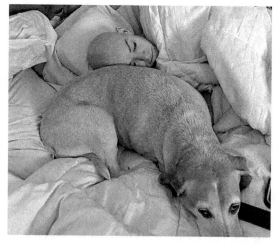

Piper took such good care of me.

course, you do. That's kind of what it's like after a bunch of mean chemotherapy treatments. Except, I wasn't taunting my opponent. I was shouting, "Chill out dude. Can't we be friends?" Apparently not. And the worst part of it is how truly appreciative I was for my cancer-killing chemo. It was ironic that the measures being taken to save my life were also destroying me at the same time. But that's how chemo works. I was fully committed to my treatment plan, but walking into FCS for round five still caused major anxiety. This was as much of a mental game as it was a physical one. The infusion went as usual and I was sent home to curl up with Piper, who had officially earned the title of "Best Dog Ever."

June 17. Monday.

At this point, I was spending most of my days lying in bed watching Netflix and sleeping. *The Walking Dead, Frasier, and* Jerry Seinfeld's *Comedians in Cars Getting Coffee* kept me occupied for months. Sure, I'd go out to get IV fluids, acupuncture, a massage, or physical therapy, but for the most part, I was either passed out or watching endless amounts of TV. After watching all of the good stuff, I even turned on the Real Housewives of some town that I can't remember. I loathe reality TV, so this may give you a little insight into how low things had become. I could only deal with it for about 20 minutes, but holy cow. I saw lots of plastic surgery and lots of shouting. It seemed like an odd way to live. Even as a noisy person, I never shout at anyone in an angry way. And I certainly wouldn't hang with a crew that was shouting at me or constantly accusing me of nefarious things. No, thank you!

During this time, Parker went to lacrosse camp for a week, so I took responsibility for dropping him off in the morning and picking him up around noon. Temperatures were near 100 degrees, so I had been pretty concerned that he stayed hydrated and wore lots of sunscreen. Normally, I take great pleasure in Florida's sticky heat. Boiling temperatures and intense humidity have always made me happy. Chemo Fitz could barely manage walking the short distance between her house and car without the heat making her sick, which was pretty aggravating. When I picked up Parker from the first day of camp, I got out of the car and stood with the other parents to watch the boys scrimmage. Parker had never played before and when I pulled up, I could hear the coaches shouting his name enthusiastically. I was really eager to see him in action and find out what he was doing so well. But I was only on the sideline for about 90 seconds before the heat started making me feel nauseous. I was trying hard to power through and watch my boy be sporty, but within a few minutes I had to retreat to my car. If I hadn't, I would have certainly passed out and caused a commotion. How lame. I just wanted to see enough to be able to lay specific praise on Parker during our drive home, but I was too weak to even spectate. It was very frustrating.

June 20. Thursday.

I was back in the air heading to Kansas City, Missouri. I still felt like crap, but I was determined as ever to do my job. This was another DC Wonder Woman Run Series race weekend, which meant another chance to sport my blue tutu with white stars and sparkly red shoes. Besides a crazy storm drenching our official merchandise tent and a bit of rain on race day, this was a really easy, drama-free weekend. The race started

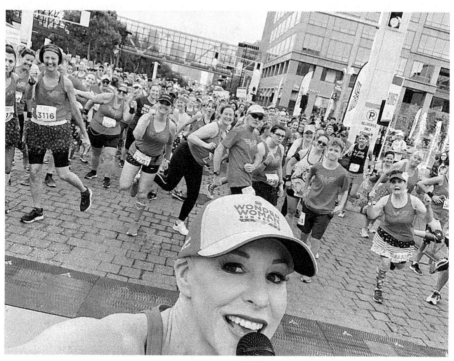

Striking a pose with my Kansas City Wonder Woman squad!

and finished in the posh Hallmark Centre and included tons of families with children. Our athletes were super energetic and an absolute delight to work with. Of note for me, I was only able to consume strawberry smoothies that weekend. That's right. Only strawberry smoothies. My fickle and angry stomach had decided to wage war on all other food products. Fortunately, my hotel was close to two food spots that made strawberry smoothies. I went through about seven of them between arrival and departure.

June 23. Sunday.

As Murphy's Law would have it, nothing about my flights home from Kansas City went as planned. One delay led to the next and that one to another. I was supposed to land in Gainesville around 2 p.m., but at 6 p.m. I was still wandering around the Atlanta airport like a zombie. My last plane wouldn't even take off until 8:30 pm. You know what they say: "When things go wrong, don't go with them." So instead of just stewing with anger I had a fantastic idea. I remembered that the Delta Sky Club in Terminal E had shower facilities. Now, in no way did I actually need a shower. But a nice hot shower sounded like a heck of a lot more fun than rotting in a chair somewhere, so off to Terminal E I went. And I am

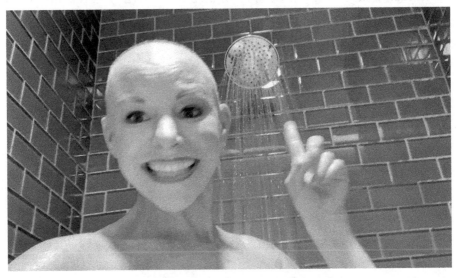

Party for one in the airport shower!

so glad I did. These shower facilities were luxurious and felt like a spa. I basically had a master bathroom to myself. It was perfectly clean, with bright red-tiled walls, lovely toiletries, fluffy towels, and a huge shower. I undressed, played music from my phone, and remained under the piping hot water for almost an hour. It was exquisite. I even stayed through some sort of airport crisis.

I was stretching and singing along to Garth Brooks when the fire alarm started buzzing. Loudly. Naked in the Delta Sky Club shower is not really where one wants to be during any sort of emergency, but there I was. Naked and not really afraid. At first I thought that I should probably get dressed and head out. But the shower felt so good and I figured that if there was a real fire, someone would probably run back yelling, "Fire" and then I'd know for sure. But if the alarm was buzzing because of an active shooter or some other evil-doer, I decided that being naked in the Delta Sky Club shower was probably a really clever place to be. What were the odds that a gun-wielding wacko would leave the main terminal, charge through the Sky Lounge and come seek the shower people out? Even if a bad guy did come to seek out the shower people, I was behind a dead-bolted door and a tiled wall. Naked in the Sky Club was actually pretty genius. Eventually, the alarm stopped buzzing and I continued enjoying my little slice of airport heaven. I never found out why the alarm was buzzing, but I didn't see anything on the news. We can just assume Delta ran out of pretzels or something. I arrived home a little before midnight.

While I would never voluntarily choose bald for myself, it does have a few bright sides. With the yuckiness that came from being sick and the constant feeling of the green alien sludge rolling around under my scalp, it was wonderful to be able to jump into the shower or bath several times a day. Having water run directly on my head was relieving. I didn't have that luxury as a long-haired lady (I also didn't have alien sludge). Not because I couldn't get my hair wet, but because getting that hair dry again was a pain in the can. The luscious locks that I loved and lost were not only long, they were also shockingly thick. It could take

*up to 45 minutes of blow-drying to get the job done, which was
not something I would have wanted to do several times a day.
Looking at the bright side of baldness, this qualified.*

June 27. Thursday.

This was a bit of a wonky day. I was flying to Fargo, North Dakota for
another DC Wonder Woman Run Series race weekend and had to take
three different flights to get there. Gainesville > Atlanta > Minneapolis
> Fargo. Now, if you fly often, you know that the more connections one
has, the more likely one will suffer delays and/or confront obstacles. This
weekend exemplified that. Getting to Atlanta was easy and boarding
my plane to Minneapolis wasn't a problem. Landing, however, became
a huge issue. About 20 minutes before my plane was supposed to touch
down in Minneapolis for my very short layover, the pilot notified us that
because of a storm, we were going to do circles in the air for a while.
About 40 minutes later, when I was guaranteed to miss my flight from
Minneapolis to Fargo, we were notified that our plane needed gas and
we were going to land in Fargo to get it. FABULOUS! What luck, right?
Wrong.

It was noon as our plane soared toward Fargo. I bragged to our flight
attendant that this situation was going to work wonders for me since
Fargo was my final destination. With a sorrowful look on her face, she let
me know that I wouldn't be able to debark in Fargo because we weren't
going to pull up to a gate. I would have to fly back to Minneapolis, debark, rebook my flight and then return to Fargo. OMG. Seriously? This
couldn't be happening. Can you imagine the mental torture involved in
this situation? I was being held hostage and I had no way to fight back. I
asked the flight attendant if she could just claim that I was being drunk
and disorderly so they'd kick me off the plane. I figured a few hours
stuck in security or Fargo jail would be far more pleasant than being
stuck in the Minneapolis airport all day. Unfortunately, she refused.

As we sat on the runway for the next hour, about six other passengers
with a final destination of Fargo started bellyaching. The flight atten-
dants pleaded our case to the pilots, who then pleaded our case to the

airport authorities. After a long wait, the airport people agreed to send a guy out, in a bright yellow vest, with a flashlight of some sort to escort us into the airport. *That was all it took? Why didn't they agree to do that right away?* I was thrilled to have escaped that plane and to be avoiding the painful situation of yo-yoing back and forth. They refused to take our luggage off the plane, but I was more than fine with retrieving it later that night.

When I checked into the hotel, my stomach was pretty miserable and all I was craving was noodle soup. One would think it would be an easy thing to attain, but it wasn't. I roamed the city streets for over an hour trying to find a restaurant that sold it. My tummy was giving me buckle-over hunger pains, but nothing else sounded edible. Finally, before I dropped dead in the streets, I stumbled across the Smiling Moose Rocky Mountain Deli, which had it on the menu. I can't tell you how happy I was to get off of my feet and finally eat. The soup tasted horrible because, like everything else I ate, it was coated with black dirt. But I was happy to have it anyway.

After napping in my hotel room for an hour or so, I dragged myself over to the Wonder Woman team dinner. It was hosted by Mark Knutson, who was also the owner of the Fargo Marathon. He's a soft-spoken leader who's creative, thoughtful, generous, and can always be found doing hard labor on race day. Dinner was tough. I really wanted to be with all of the fabulous people I was working with, but I was drained and my stomach was a mess. It's a strange experience to be both starving and unable to eat at the same time. The company was superb, and I worked pretty hard to engage, but I was definitely less chatty than I would have liked to have been. Toward the end of our meal, race director Beth and her sweetpea hubby John Hamrick came over to check on me. John, whom I also became close friends with, pitched in with operations and photography, but was mostly known for his bear hugs. They said I could be honest with them about how I was feeling, and I knew that they were genuinely concerned. I considered them both dear friends and in any other scenario, I would have come clean. If I had been truthful, they would have undoubtedly responded in a very compassionate way. The downside to all of that would have been me falling apart, and sobbing that night was not on my to-do list. Admitting how sick I felt wasn't going to boost my mental health either. When I returned home from Fargo, I was headed straight in for mean chemo #6 and the thought of that was weighing heavily on my mind. I needed to stay tough and not relent to the crap that was trying to crush me, both physically and mentally. I had a lot of work to do that weekend and any faint break in my armor would have diminished my abilities. Instead of telling Beth and John the truth, I smiled and told them I was just a little tired.

After Mark gave the crew quirky Fargo-themed shirts, we all went our separate ways. My shirt had a big "Uffda!" on the front. In Fargo lingo, Uffda is associated with relief, surprise, and a few other feelings. Dontcha know? Folks from Fargo talk a little funny, which is part of their charm. As my colleagues walked toward a pub or to relax at the hotel, I walked my pathetic booty a few blocks over to a convenience store to buy some tolerable food for the weekend. Yogurt cups and cans of noodle soup were some of the things I took back with me. It was getting dark and this bald chick was roaming the streets of Fargo alone, looking for gas station food. Oof! Quite often, people express how envious they are of my glamorous travel life. That always makes me think of times like these. Sure, there are a ton of fancy hotels and restaurants, but on occasion, I'm eating gas station food and feeling grateful for it.

When I got back to the hotel, my stomach was so volatile that I ended up spending half of the night on the bathroom floor. Why do we do that? I mean, I know it's so we're not far from the toilet, but for some reason, the bathroom floor feels super comfortable when I'm sick. When I had a stomach bug as a kid, I'd sleep on the bathroom floor. When I had too much fun in college, I'd sleep on the bathroom floor. I'm pretty sure that it would never feel delightful on a normal day, but on sick days, the bathroom floor is the comfiest coziest place in the world.

June 28. Friday.

When I woke up and forced my body off of the cold and hard-yet-comfy bathroom floor, I took a long hot shower, enjoyed a fancy gas station yogurt, and put on my favorite Wonder Woman tutu. Our race expo was held inside the Fargo Civic Center, and being indoors was a fantastic reward for me. I was able to comfortably make my announcements while interacting with our athletes, without heat becoming a factor. When I needed a break, I just sat on my stage and made announcements from a chair. Uffda!

June 29. Saturday.

We started off the morning with our Wonder Woman trivia and costume contests. I love interacting with our participants because they are usually very gregarious and extroverted people. Shy folks don't tend to voluntarily get on a stage, so the personalities of our costumed contestants are traditionally bold. We laughed a lot as they answered questions and everyone oohed and aahed over their attire. During the contests the arena started to fill up with thousands of people. You see, we were actually launching the races from inside the building. That was something I hadn't done before and I found the experience pretty neat. The energy was combustible and, because the arena walls trapped the crowd's shouts and cheers, everything felt twice as loud. I started the 10K first while the 5K athletes cheered from the bleachers. This was really cool for both the athletes giving and receiving the support. Once they took off through a massive open corner of the arena, the 5K crew moved down to start their race. In the crowd was Amy Roux, one of my favorite sarcastic mommy friends from Gainesville who moved to Sioux Falls, South Dakota many years ago. She and her 12-year-old daughter, Nadia, drove in to see me and run. I tell you, nothing is more flattering than when people get into a car or board a plane and travel far from the comfort of their home to see me. What?! For me? I've had a few close friends do it, but I've also had tons of people I barely know who have traveled across the country to run a race specifically because I was the announcer. It's incredible.

We ended up with a bizarre timing/sound issue at the indoor finish line, so I spent much of the morning outside welcoming runners and walkers home. At one point, I even took a seat right next to a giant dumpster, with my microphone to do my job. I know you're impressed with my fanciness, but sometimes you gotta do what you gotta do! More importantly, every moment I spent with these athletes made me feel better. Not perfect, but they energized me and used their powers of awe-someness to help me forget what was going wrong with my body. It was a fantastic gift they likely had no idea they were giving. The people of Fargo were magnificent, and *doncha know*, I would go back any day to make noise for them.

Post-race, Amy and Nadia drove back to the arena to pick me up, so we could go to lunch together. I was still not feeling right, but nothing was going to keep me from quality time with the Rouxs. On the way to lunch, I saw my first real tumbleweed blowing across some train tracks and since I'd only really seen them before in cartoons, I found it pretty neat. We parked on the side of a pizza place for lunch and went inside to eat and catch up. They're both so smart and snarky, and we had a won-derful time. Leaving lunch was more than a little exciting. A crazy storm was blowing through town causing traffic barriers and other large debris to fly through the streets. We literally had to run to the car ducking and dodging to avoid being hit. Uffda!

Our entire team went over to Mark's house that evening for a get-to-gether. It was an easy night and I was happy to hang with everyone with-out having to put in too much effort. I'm fortunate to collaborate with such lovely people. Every last person on our DC Wonder Woman Run Series team was a gem and we all got along so well. I was the first to leave the party because I had to be up outrageously early to fly home — 3 a.m. for my 5:10 a.m. flight, to be exact. What idiot booked this flight? Ummm. This idiot. I did.

Fitzness Log

Once again, there was absolutely no deliberate exercise for me. Other than stretching in the shower, all I could do was rest and recover. Push-ing that envelope was only going to land me back in the hospital. I often wondered how regular able-bodied people could neglect their health and treat exercise like it was a punishment, when all I wanted to do was feel well enough to be athletic again.

Chapter 7

Despair and Determination

July 1. Monday.

Getting ready for my final round of the mean chemo was like preparing to walk the green mile. I was dead-tired, suffering from horrendous tummy issues and millions of other wicked side effects. I still had most of my muscles and lashes, but every other part of my poor body, inside and out, had been at least partially destroyed. While many people innocently kept asking, "Are you excited for your last chemo?" or suggesting that things would be over after this sixth round, what they didn't understand is that chemo just kicked off the suffering. It was the catalyst. The thought of feeling even worse, was beyond daunting. If you've ever seen the old movie *Misery*, you'll remember the hobbling scene where James Caan's character wakes up strapped to a bed with a wooden block affixed between his feet. His captor, played by Kathy Bates, wants to ensure he won't escape, so she takes a massive swing with a sledgehammer and breaks both of his ankles. It was a disturbing scene that made almost everyone squirm. It was hideous. From my perspective, asking me if I was looking forward to my final round of mean chemo was equivalent to asking if I was excited about being hobbled again. I wasn't.

As I signed in to see Dr. Gordan, I was given a short questionnaire to fill out, which was a bit of a psychiatric checkup. It asked questions to gauge levels of fatigue, functionality, motivation, hopelessness, etc. Apparently, my responses set off the alarm with Dr. Gordan. It was unusual having him offer antidepressants or counseling because, "Hey. I'm Fitz Koehler. I'm impenetrable!" Well, apparently not. While I wasn't going to harm myself, I was definitely depressed and mentally beaten down. I cried all the freaking time. I cried because things hurt. I cried from exhaustion, fatigue, nerves, and more. Life had snowballed out of control, and my levels of stress were immeasurable. And being on some sort of psychological watch list did not thrill me. I loved Dr. Gordan for his care and professionalism, but I resented this nonsense affecting my mental health. I did not take him up on his offers for support, but I definitely appreciated that he made an effort. He also offered to postpone my treatment for a week if I needed a break. I refused. I was on a mission to massacre every single cancer cell in my body, without giving them even the slightest chance to survive or spread. I also wanted to get this phase over with. One more round of the mean stuff, he promised. And then I should start feeling better.

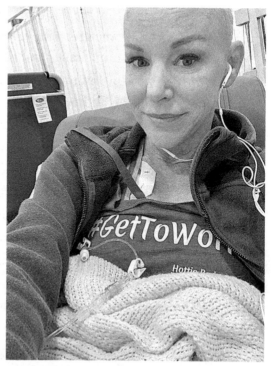

Receiving my final round of mean chemo.
Wrapped in my baby blanket.

Once again, I headed back for some quality time with Lilly. My infusion went as usual on this sixth and final day of mean chemo: I arrived, got hooked up, and did my best to sleep through as much of the day as possible.

By this point, my stomach seemed to know exactly how it was supposed to respond to each particular drug and began reacting to each as they were being delivered. Taxotere in — stomach contents out! I didn't have that happen during the first chemo, but as my treatment progressed, the side effects would kick in almost immediately. My poor tummy. After having my final Neulasta device attached to my very sore and bruised arms, I was pleased that Piper had her tushy ready for my head so that we could get some sleep. Did I feel relieved that the mean chemo treatments were over? I don't know. Maybe. It's hard to feel any sort of relief when you're in the thick of it.

July 4. Thursday.

The great gift of chemo #6 was that I had 11 full days at home before embarking on my next flight. That was a huge relief. And as any sane person would suggest, my game-plan moving forward from nightmare #6 *should* have been to lie flat on my back in bed, watch crappy TV, and avoid the world. However, since I have close to zero common sense, I had one big thing to do between this point and my next visit to the airport. I was hosting a party for about 100 people three days after my final mean chemo. I know. I'm an idiot. Fourth of July is a big deal for my very patriotic family, and we celebrate it every year with a massive bash at our home. It's a bring-a-dish style gathering that starts at 4 p.m. and ends around 10 p.m. Our regular-sized home fills with all sorts of important people from all aspects of our lives, and we absolutely love it. We've been doing it since Ginger was one year old, and I was committed to not allowing cancer to take this awesome annual experience away from my family, my friends, and myself.

Rob and the kids were going to do all of the prep-work: yard work, house cleaning, decorating, shopping, and set-up. My only obligation was to email the invites and take part in the party as much or as little as I could. That's basically how things turned out. I stayed in bed until our first guest arrived, and then I got up, got dressed, and showed my face. It's all a bit of a blur, but I remember going from room to room to sit with friends and try to be a gracious host. Everyone was concerned about me. I did my best to pretend everything was fine and encourage them to have fun. My house was packed. Usually, folks hang out in our yard too, but we were having our typical Florida summer storms and outside wasn't an option. It was loud and crowded with kids running everywhere and the food spread was incredible. Besides the traditional barbecued meats and sides we provided, our tables were overflowing with homemade masterpieces including pizza rolls, black bean dip, mac n' cheese, egg rolls, chicken wing dip, spinach dip, veggie platters, fruit salads, and an infinite amount of desserts. I really wanted to partake, but when I put a few of my favorites on a plate and took a bite, it all tasted horrible. Everything was still covered in black dirt, and I wanted to punch my stupid taste buds! I don't know about you, but I absolutely adore bring-a-dish events where you get to try everyone's favorite creations. My friends and neighbors make some of the best food, and I was pissed that I was being deprived of enjoying it. I wanted to ask everyone to bring back their dishes in a few months when I could taste things properly again. But I didn't. I actually lied to everyone and told them everything was yummy. I didn't want to disappoint anyone. Even though I wasn't able to bounce around as usual, everyone seemed to have a fantastic time. I intermixed low-key socialization with hiding out in my room with Piper for some rest. I probably attended almost 50% of the party, and that was just fine. One of our claims to fame is a Disney-esque fireworks show. As the sun sets, our guests head out to our front lawn with chairs and desserts. Under strict supervision, we start with little handheld sparklers for the kids, which they go bonkers over. Once several hundred of them have been lit, we launch simple single screamers up in the air. After that, we continue to light up the night's sky with all sorts of dazzling, colorful, and noisy explosions. The same kind your city likely deploys on the Fourth and New Year's Eve. Also, when I say "we" do fireworks I don't mean Rob and I. A few of our buddies who love playing with fireworks, man the show. We've been doing this for so many years that someone actually built a sturdy stand with canisters to keep things safe and ensure the fireworks go up instead of twisting to the side. Many of our neighbors do the same thing, which makes for colorful explosions no matter where you look. I can comfortably say that my front lawn is one of the most fabulous places to be in Florida on the Fourth of July. Why go get stuck in traffic for some city event and use porta-potties when you can chill at the Koehler Mansion with real bathrooms, yummy food, and a magnificent show? You wouldn't. Not if you're on the guest list, at least. I passed out in bed with Piper before 10 p.m., but our home didn't clear out until 11 p.m. I physically struggled to get through it all, but if I could go back in time and change it, I wouldn't.

This was an ENORMOUS victory for me. I know cancer wasn't some asshole with a personal vendetta against me, but sometimes that's how it felt. That's why continuing to do the big things in life felt like real triumphs. I don't appreciate anyone or anything taking my personally-declared essentials: my life, my experiences, my work, my people. This party mattered for all of those reasons. Was it insane to host a party for 100 people three days after my sixth round of mean chemo? Absolutely. Was it still awesome? You're damn right, it was. Patriotic party point awarded to ... Fitz Koehler!

When I wasn't going in for IV fluids, I spent the week lying in bed. I was weak and fatigued with an insurmountable list of other side effects. And on top of that, my final race announcing gig of the summer was coming up. I needed to recharge. My kids were preparing for camp without my support, and while I was sad about not being helpful, I was impressed that they could work together to do so on their own. Even though I felt like I was really likely to survive my bout with breast cancer, my mortality was continuously on my mind. I was perpetually working to make sure my kids knew important bits of information and learned vital skills in case I wasn't around anymore. They were little things, but they mattered to me. I remember Parker being argumentative when I forced him to learn how to cook his own chicken breast on the stove. He wasn't in the mood for it, but he had no idea I was thinking, "You need to know how to cook in case I die!" I didn't tell him that at the time, but I think if he knew why I was pushing the issue, he would have been more receptive. Oh well. Kids are kids. I also urged Rob to teach Ginger and Parker how to mow the lawn and fix things around the house. We are strong parents who've raised wonderful little humans, but we could do better teaching them the skills they'll need to manage their own home someday.

July 5. Friday.

I had definitely hit the point where every millimeter of my body had been harmed in some way, and I looked every bit as foul as I felt. I also had developed a really nasty odor. Believe it or not, my fingernails started to stink. In fact, I think they were actually rotting. I discovered this while doing something relatively simple like scratching my nose. Can you imagine how appalling it would be to have rotting fingernails? It came out of the blue, and there was virtually nothing I could do to correct it. I washed my hands a billion times with lemon-scented soap and water, ineffectively slathered on antibacterial gels, and tried all sorts of yummy-smelling lotions to remove the stench. Nothing worked. Nights and naps were disrupted because I always sleep on my side, with my hands underneath my face, and the odor was unbearable. I ended up having to put small towels or pillows between my hands and face to get comfy. I eventually got some sort of antifungal products to put on my nails, which I think helped, but this delightful phenomenon lasted for about two weeks. Again, while the world was sending me messages about how easy I was making this look, parts of me were literally rotting. I was sick, sore, exhausted, bald, weak, and emotionally fragile, with yellow, bumpy, short, and stinky nails.

July 12. Friday.

Same airport. Same stupid look on my face when saying good-bye to Rob. I was flying to Denver, Colorado for yet another DC Wonder Woman Run Series event. I wasn't in any shape to travel, but I wasn't following any rules. I was going to earn a living doing what I loved, and nothing was going to stop me. And even though the expression on my face was stupid, my actual face was infinitely more stupid. All of the eyelashes on my right eye had fallen out. That's right. Just the right eye. On the left side, however, there were about 20 lashes left. They looked as if they were taking some strange stand as if they were protecting the Alamo. And to exaggerate the disparity, my lashes still contained the lash extensions

I'd been wearing for months. Leftie was super fabulous, while rightie was straight up bald. Yeah. I looked absurd. To try to compensate for the unevenness, I glued strip lashes to both eyes. Strip lashes were tricky enough to attach under normal circumstances, but without any lashes for them to sit on top of, they were near impossible. It's hard to describe what it's like being trapped in a strange bald head and having freaky uneven lashes. It's the kind of thing that makes you want to have a tantrum. In fact, lying on the ground, kicking and screaming, and flailing probably would have been seriously satisfying. But that would have exhausted me, so instead, I just breathed deeply and tried to remain dignified.

If you've ever seen the movie Toy Story, you might remember a strange little mutant toy named Babyface who was created by the mean kid, Sid. Babyface was basically a baby doll head that was attached to robotic spider legs. His right eye was completely missing, but his left eye was big and blue with beautiful lashes. It was just like me! First Shrek, and now this. While conjuring up these animated characters stemmed from my sarcastic sense of humor, I actually identified with them. The correlations were kind of funny, but only because there was a lot of truth behind them. And while laughing about my steadily deteriorating appearance, photos of the old me would regularly pop up and I would think, "I was so pretty!" That would sting a bit. Looking like Shrek made me laugh. Looking back at the girl I used to be, was bittersweet. I wasn't really looking forward to standing on stages all weekend looking like Babyface. Thank goodness for sunglasses!

Unsurprisingly, I arrived in Denver feeling drained. My hotel was in the heart of the downtown area, just a few blocks away from our start and finish line. A team dinner was held that night but I skipped it in lieu of unsuccessfully roaming the streets trying to find some noodle soup. My poor planning was becoming a real bore. If I had an intelligent bone in my body, I would have started traveling with cans of Campbell's Soup, but apparently, I did not.

Added to my list of weird stuff to pack:
- Nail Fungus Drops

- Campbell's Soup
- 75,000 prescriptions "just in case"
- List of chemo drugs I'm on "just in case"

July 13. Saturday.

Our expo was held in a big beautiful park, right in between the State Capital and City Hall. The set-up was lovely, but oof! The combination of elevation (one mile high) and 99-degree temperatures made for a rough day. This Floridian tends to work best at sea level, and Little Miss Chemotherapy was not responding well to the heat. It was the first event that I truly didn't make a major effort to mingle with our participants. Usually, I'd flit around the booths like a butterfly getting to know our runners while answering questions and helping them shop for race day outfits. Instead, I did a lot of sitting on my stage making announcements in the shade. A perk of that was all of the local vagrants who chose to demonstrate their special dancing skills for me when they liked a particular song. On occasion, some would shout profanities at me, but our crew would offer a little support, and the wackiness would subside. The elements were oppressive, so halfway through my 6-hour workday, I took 30 minutes to escape to a nearby McDonald's. Leaving an event is unheard of for me, but I needed some air conditioning and a cold milkshake to hit the spot. I also asked to leave early, which I have simply never done before. I was supposed to finish at 6 p.m., but around 4 p.m. I started feeling like I wasn't going to make it. I asked Beth if I could leave a little early (meaning 5:30 p.m.) and she sweetly told me to go back to my hotel right away. I tried to argue, but she didn't want to risk losing me for race day if I pushed too hard. Her logic was inarguable, and I headed back to my hotel. On the short five-block walk, I buckled over quite a few times, thinking I might get sick. I had to stop and rest quite frequently as well. Even though the distance was small, I should have grabbed an Uber. Making it back to my room safely was a relief.

When I arrived, I threw off my clothes and went straight into the shower to sit on the floor and let water pour over me. I was toast. My body felt like it was disintegrating and my lashes were driving me insane. As I sat there, soaked, I systematically pulled out all of the lash extensions on my left eye. Well, I thought I was only pulling out the extensions, but any remaining real lashes also fell out. Crap. I was so disappointed to have failed on two of my three mini-goals. Remember? I wanted to keep my muscles, keep my lashes, and never spend a night in the hospital. Dang it. I was happy to have some symmetry back on my face, but I quickly went from Babyface to Voldemort. You know. The creepy bald villain from Harry Potter.

July 14. Sunday.

This would prove to be my closest call for trouble while announcing. That morning, I had the pleasure of having my dear friend, Creigh Kelley as my co-announcer. Creigh is a Denver resident and Vietnam veteran, who has a magnificent history in the running community as a race director, race announcer, agent, ambassador, and athlete. He is a sweet soul, who has survived his own scary bout with cancer. I've been grateful for his support throughout my treatment, and I was proud to stand next to him as he looked dy-no-mite in his tight white announcing pants (this is a real thing). We started off the day with our traditional trivia and costume contests, which were relaxed, enjoyable, and very entertaining. But as soon as we finished, it was time to hustle over to our start line stage, maybe 100 yards away. Not very far for the average Jane, but I was semi-dehydrated, very depleted, and not in shape for moving quickly in the Mile High City. When we arrived, I was pretty winded, but also invigorated by the thousands of people who had converged on the area for the 10K and 5K starts.

Since I usually do not work with a co-announcer at our DC Wonder Woman Run Series events, our sound team was prepared with only one microphone. That made it incredibly challenging to co-host an event where casual banter is key. Creigh and I passed the mic back and forth for a while, but once I had to start getting through the nitty-gritty nuts and bolts of important stuff specific to these races, Creigh decided to go set up at the finish line. That totally made sense and was probably the right thing to do, but a few minutes after he left, I started going downhill. Nausea struck, I was struggling to breathe properly, and everything looked kind of yellow. I remember staring out at the crowd of thou-

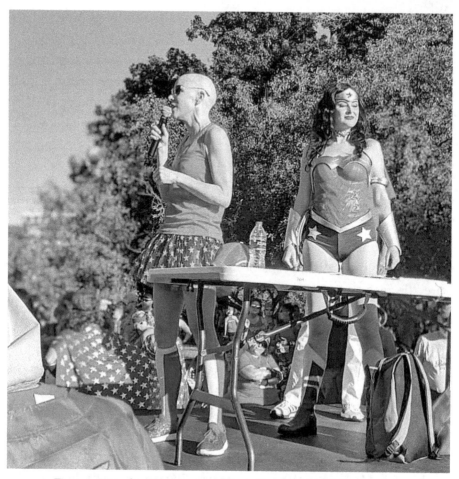

Denver Wonder Woman start line. Grateful I didn't pass out.
Jay Sutherland/Sport Photo Group

sands thinking, "Please don't pass out. Please don't pass out!" Denver was spinning. And then I looked down below my stage and saw that it was surrounded by concrete and the words in my head became "Don't break bones! Don't break bones! Don't break bones!" I was losing control quickly.

I don't know if you can call it a miracle, but I was only able to keep my composure because of Kent Kolstad. He's the president of Livewire, which provides all audio and video services for our events. About 10 seconds before I hit the ground, Kent randomly showed up with a snack and drink for me. Fluids and calories were exactly what I needed. Had

160

he not done so, I'm about 99% positive I would have passed out. Grateful for his gifts, I took the opportunity to refuel, re-energize, and shut up so the crowd could enjoy the music and each other. I've thanked him a few times since, but I still don't think Kent understands the magnitude of how big a save he made. Can you imagine how awful it would have been if I'd toppled off of my stage in front of all of those people? Yikes! I just narrowly escaped that happening.

After surviving what turned out to be a wild start line experience, I slowly meandered over to the finish line, where I was more than happy to let Creigh do his thing. He hung out in the chute and greeted runners while I sat on a chair in the shade and welcomed them by name using our laptop. Denver had put a fork in me. That was the first, and will remain the last, time I ever stay seated at a finish line.

My special people from this weekend included my Hottie Anthony Wilk who delayed his move from Denver to Arizona to stay in town to see me. He's lost over 90 pounds using my Exact Formula for Weight Loss, and I loved getting to spend some quality time with him. He ran in a custom-made "Wonder Woman Fitz Strong" shirt that touched my heart. I also met a fellow breast cancer patient, Megan Price, after she finished the 10K with a shiny bald head. I'll tell you what. Megan was beautiful and sunny, and I completely admired her ability to run during treatment. We had the exact opposite responses to chemo, and I was so happy for her. I've been following her progress since, and she is doing great.

Denver was uniquely difficult, but I took solace knowing that if things went as planned, my health would never be that bad for a race weekend again. I wasn't completely done with treatment, but I was done with the mean stuff, and things had to get easier, right?

July 16. Tuesday.

After spending an extra day in Denver to rest, I took an uneventful flight to Orlando. Instead of going straight home to Gainesville, I was re-routing so that I would be able to watch Ginger perform and compete at her summer cheerleading camp at UCF (University of Central Florida). Rob's best friend, Scott Hartog, picked me up from the airport and brought me to his and his wife's beautiful home to spend the night. Oh, what a night it turned out to be! I kicked things off by sobbing in their living room in a rare and pathetic emotional outburst. Sure, I had every reason to blubber, but I still hated doing so. Even though I consider them family, the breakdown was embarrassing. They made a wonderful home-cooked meal for Rob, who had arrived by car, and me, but I left the table without eating because I just couldn't handle being awake or upright anymore.

The Hartogs have a big cozy bed in their guest suite. But instead of utilizing that cozy bed, I ended up spending most of the night tossing and turning on the floor. I'm still not sure why sleeping on the floor is my top choice when my tummy turns, but for some reason, it feels far better to me than any sort of luxurious mattress. Around 2 a.m., my stomach was screaming for food because I hadn't eaten dinner, so I crept out to raid their fridge. Unfortunately, Scott and Leslie were on a serious health kick, and I couldn't find anything other than fruits and vegetables. I was pleased to see them making great choices, but cranky tummies do not like that kind of roughage. I was hoping for something bland like crackers, but I couldn't find anything even remotely close. After digging in their cabinets for a few minutes, I was relieved to find one chocolate doughnut and I brought it back to my room. I took one bite of it and then passed out on the floor, still holding it. I woke up with the rest of the doughnut smeared all over my arms and face. The life of Voldemort was not very glamorous! There were many low points on this journey, but as I stood in the bathroom and gazed into the mirror cleaning the chocolate goo off of my face, head, and arms, I was pretty disappointed with who I'd become.

July 17. Wednesday.

I still felt lousy as we drove to Ginger's cheerleading competition, but nothing was going to stop me from seeing my athletic little lady perform. Cheerleading for her high school has been so beneficial to her. The sport is fun and she's surrounded by lovely teammates. Plus, her coach, Teameika Trueluck, is the ultimate role model. She's not only effectively leading cheerleading squads, she's also raising three delightful daughters, and is a Sheriff's Deputy and the high school's resource officer. She's strong, moral, thoughtful, and trustworthy. The team had spent a week at camp and this was the grand finale. I wanted to be there, and Ginger wanted me to be there too. She showed her appreciation by bounding over during breaks to give me hugs and kisses. Unsurprisingly, her sweetness made me feel much better. Ginger and her team crushed their performance and Rob and I cheered obnoxiously. In fact, all of the teams competing were exciting to watch. It made me crazy proud to be a cheer mom.

I'm going to share a bit of advice. If you ever have a sick or injured loved one insist on going to special events, even though you've offered them the opportunity to stay home, please accept their wishes. Even when I felt like hell, I was happy to be taking part in life. I can't imagine what it's like to be terminal, but I can guess that dying folks want to get the most out of whatever time they have left. If sitting in an arena sick as hell was a positive for me, then I bet others may feel that way too.

And on that note, I want to talk about living with a terminal disease. I'm more than grateful that my prognosis was a good one, but I had some awful insight into what it might be like if things were different. At some point, I was so sick, tired, and sad that I was able to identify with why terminal patients stop pursuing life-extending treatments. In the past, I'd not been able to truly comprehend why anyone would purposely stop trying to kill their cancer and just resolve to accept death. I'm a girl who wants every single moment and memory I can get. The thought of giving up never seemed reasonable. But during my own experience, I finally understood. My treatment was destroying me. It was hard to eat, sleep, and be awake. My stomach never stopped screaming. My head, quads, throat, hands, fingernails, toenails, and every other body part hurt. I cried all the time and experienced true despair. I endured it all because I was promised a cure. But what if I wasn't? What if I was being destroyed with no long-term benefit? I might have stopped showing up. I didn't like being able to identify with people in that situation. It hurt my heart for all of those I've loved and lost to cancer who had made the agonizing decision to stop treatment.

Since I was done with work travel for the next two months and because Ginger and Parker were both away at camp for the next week or so, I was finally able to get some real rest. That helped me start turning the corner on the mean chemo. It was perfect timing that Denver was my last race of the summer. I have faith I could have pulled off another miracle on the microphone, but I was re-

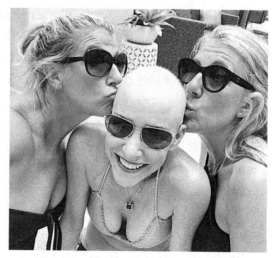

Head kisses from Nicole Bodlack and Jennifer Hawthorne.

lieved that I didn't have to. A few bright spots as I took things super easy included Parker surprising me with a quick trip home from camp. Sure, it'd only been about nine days since I'd last seen him, but our reunion looked a little like he'd just returned from war. His hugs have been one of my greatest sources of comfort since he was born, so I latched on and didn't let go. Another high point was when Jennifer Jaroneczyk Hawthorne, one of my favorite friends from high school, flew down from New York to spend time with me. She, Nicole Zimmerman Bodlack, and I all grew up together, and our time together was absolutely medicinal. It'd been a long time since I'd had some easy laughs with girlfriends, and it felt like a breath of fresh air. We sat in the shade by Nicole's pool and chatted for hours. The picture we took of them kissing my bald head is one I'll cherish forever.

My friends have been pretty remarkable throughout this experience. And I'll repeat what I've said before: I have been overwhelmed by kindness, generosity, and support. And I've also been underwhelmed by the lack of action from others. I've had a core group of friends with me for decades that I'll put in the category of people that I would drop anything for. And I had confidence they would do the same for me. Most of my ride or die friends showed up. They called, visited, texted, and let me know that they were thinking of me and loved me a lot. Seeing their names pop up on my phone with a text always put a smile on my face. And then there were other close friends who did none of the above. It's totally okay, and I still love them, but I was definitely surprised. I have a strict policy of not expecting anything from anyone because that's one of the best ways to avoid disappointment. If you expect nothing and get nothing, there can never be a problem. However, I had *cancer.* A call or a text from those best friends would have been appreciated. I didn't expect them to drop everything or do anything for me, but a few check-ins would have been great. My advice for anyone with a close friend going through something like this is to simply be there. If you're nearby, offer help or visit. If you're far, send a text or card to let them know you care. Little gestures like these do not go unnoticed. In fact, I had a few sweet pals who regularly sent messages that said, "You don't have to respond. Just know I love you." Those were perfect since I was often too drained to reply. Overall, I was blessed with a lot of love and support. My idiot cancer certainly inspired *some* goodness.

While I'm blessed with an endless amount of friends and fans, I'm not universally loved. It's charming that some people think I hang the moon, but not everyone feels the same. I have had quite a few people who disregarded me over the years make major U-turns since my diagnosis. There are individuals who have turned their anti-Fitz attitudes upside down and become some of my most vocal supporters. I'm happy with the extra love and friendship, but I would like to know what went on in their heads when they decided to put me back on their good list. Some Gainesville locals who had stopped communicating with me for years (not even a hello) were suddenly seeking me out to tell me how much they were rooting for me. *Shrugs* I'll take friendliness over awkward avoidance any day.

Another fascinating about-face came from the wife of one of my male runner friends. In the past, she didn't want him to chat or take post-race photos with me. I thought it was odd because her husband and I had nothing but a race day friendship, as I do with thousands of others. We were not flirty or inappropriate at all, but I understood that some people are more possessive than others. Her marriage. Her rules. However, once I became sick and bald, she changed her mind. The two of them now seek me out to chat me up, and he has full permission to loiter with me in any way he chooses. I guess the absence of my long blonde hair suddenly made me a good, non-threatening person? Neat! I truly like the couple, but their history of flip-flopping on me has been bewildering. On the other side, I know for a fact that a few of the typical mean girls I've dealt with in the past were hoping cancer would kill me quickly. And that's okay too.

July 18. Thursday.

After six rounds of the mean chemo, I went in for a PET scan. PET scans take images of everything between the top of your head and the middle of your thighs. Mine was looking for cancer. It would show us if my tumor and lymph nodes had shrunk or grew, if the cancer disappeared, or if it had spread to other parts of my body. I was really hoping for some uplifting news because I needed it. To prepare for the test, I was instructed not to consume any sugars, carbohydrates, or caffeine the day prior. And I was told I couldn't have anything at all the morning of. It wasn't awesome to deal with, but I hated food anyway and my appointment was early, so I don't recall it being too much of a burden. I arrived about an hour before my scan, at which point the radiology therapist injected some sort of sugar and nuclear fluid combo into my veins. Apparently, since sugar feeds cancer, the injected fluid would go straight to any of my cancer cells and make them light up for the camera. Unlike the MRI, this scan was fairly easy. I laid flat on a table while a short cylindrical scanner rotated around me and took images of my body. I was able to keep a claustrophobic freakout at bay because my head stuck out most of the time. It took about 20 minutes and then I was free to leave. Still sick, weak, and pathetic, I walked out and received a big hug from Rob. He quietly explained to me that during the scan, the radiology tech came out to ask him exactly where my cancer was. When Rob told him that it was in my left breast, the tech explained that he couldn't see anything at all. It was wonderful news, but I took it with a grain of salt because only the actual radiologist could make a proper diagnosis. I was pretty calm about that interaction until I got halfway down the stairs on the way out of the building and practically collapsed sobbing. Could it be? Was I actually cancer-free? Again, cancer had burdened me with endless amounts of stress. This potentially good news hit me like a ton of bricks.

Sadly, the official radiology report would eventually come in and correctly state that there was still "mild FDG activity" in my breast and lymph nodes. That meant that the nuclear fluid concoction caused some sort of seeable activity and cancer was still present. But at least it wasn't anywhere else.

July 22. Monday.

Chemo. Again. Round #7. Sure, the six rounds of mean chemo were behind me, but I still had to do eight more rounds of Herceptin. Then there was a change of plans. Because of new and changing research, Dr. Gordan explained that it would be better for me to receive both Herceptin and Perjeta for the next eight rounds. This left me petrified. Perjeta was one of the chemo drugs I'd received during the mean six, and every time I referenced my tummy issues in the infusion room, the nurses would blame them on Perjeta. How was I going to continue with tummy issues for months on end? I couldn't bear it anymore. Dr. Gordan calmly explained that we removed about 80% of the toxicity I was being given and that I should be okay. I was panicked, but he also explained that Perjeta would give me an extra few percent chances of thwarting reoccurrence. I decided to trust him and go forth because, quite frankly, I would do anything to prevent my cancer from coming back. On a nice note, instead of being at the chemo place all damn day, I was now able to go in and leave after two-ish hours. And, moving forward, the violent stomach bug style issues did not re-emerge. Dr. Gordan, the wizard, was right once again.

My six months of baldness brought me lots of interesting comparisons. Apparently, I looked a lot like some famous women and I thought I'd share the Top 10 List of my chemo doppelgangers.

- Annie Lenox
- Sinead O'Connor
- Katy Perry
- Grace Jones
- PINK
- Bald Britney Spears - Sans the umbrella
- G.I. Jane
- Bald Lady from Star Trek
- Bald Barbie
- Noisy Mannequin - This was my favorite and courtesy of my BFF Kristi Hill

July 30. Tuesday.

Surgery day. It was finally time to physically remove any remnants of my jackass cancer cells, and I was eager to get rid of them. Though I was fully confident that my surgeon, Dr. Peter Sarantos, would do an excellent job, I kept encouraging him to remove as few lymph nodes as possible. The more he removed from my armpit region, the more likely I would end up with lymphedema, which could yield chronic swelling of my arm. My great aunt had a full mastectomy for breast cancer when I was a kid, and my grandma always referenced her "sausage arm." Terrible, I know. But I couldn't get that out of my head. I didn't want a sausage arm! Dr. Sarantos continued to tell me that he would only take what was necessary to get rid of my cancer, but that the cancer removal trumped lymphedema concerns. That made sense, but I still nudged.

Surgery day did not go as I'd hoped. To make a long story short, I was scheduled to have surgery at 10 a.m., so I arrived at the hospital around 5 a.m. I purposely took an early surgical appointment because of the food restrictions. I wouldn't be allowed to eat or drink 10 hours before my surgery and I knew that starvation would make me miserable. I also insisted on a morning appointment, because in general, my very volatile stomach could only handle tiny bits of food at a time. This meant there was no way I could eat enough before midnight to hold me over until the afternoon. In fact, since I started chemo, I would often get up in the middle of the night to have a snack. Much like a baby needed a bottle, I needed calories every few hours. And much like a baby, a full tummy would put me back to sleep. If I was scheduled for an afternoon surgery, I would have said, "No thank you" and waited for a date in which a morning slot was available.

In one of the most infuriating experiences of my entire cancer battle, my doctor's nurse pushed the surgery back to 3:30 p.m. She did so at the last minute and without telling me. The change happened some time between our 6 p.m. confirmation call and my 10 a.m. appointment. I was pissed. And I didn't find out about the schedule change until after I was basically locked in from undergoing the preliminary procedures from the morning.

First of all, my IV was already set up, and that's never something I want to have an instant replay of. Second, I had been wheeled across the hospital to have some sort of nuclear goo injected into my areola — yes — they put a handful of needles into my areola, the fun little circle around my nipple. This was to make the lymph nodes more easily visible to my surgeon. The fortitude required to lay there and allow Dr. Means (his actual name) to do that was substantial. Lastly, the hospital radiologist had already inserted a huge barb into the tumor in my boob while locating it via ultrasound. The purpose of the barb was so that Dr. Sarantos could easily follow it to my tumor. That barb went inside my boob, but also stuck out of my boob. So to protect the rest of me from the external end of the barb, they covered it with a foam coffee cup and taped it to me. I wish I was kidding. So, there I was, sitting in a hospital room, starving, with my preposterous boob cup. I was eager to get things going and then I was told that I would be stuck waiting almost six extra hours.

As delightful as I try to be in most scenarios, I wanted to freaking kill someone. Locked in that little hospital room, with all sorts of sharp things stuck in me, and my stomach screaming. I was livid. Have you heard of *hangry*? That doesn't even begin to describe it. After all of the suffering and misery I'd endured as a result of cancer, this particular agony was negligently induced by a medical professional. I promise you, I like that nurse a lot. I really do. But, I could have strangled her. I paced around like a caged lion for hours, cursing alone and out loud. Poor Rob really wanted to help, but I wouldn't let him or anyone else speak. I was too furious and listening to anyone talk just pissed me off even more. I seriously contemplated kicking holes in the walls, but I kept pacing and mumbling expletives instead. My blood still boils as I retell the tale.

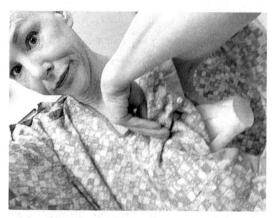

Proof I had a foam coffee cupped taped to me. What the hell?!

I had a stern talk with the nurse who screwed me over. I let her know that her actions were unprofessional and that she should have informed me about the schedule change immediately. I reminded her that her poor decisions added to the suffering of an already-punished cancer patient and that after a miserable time with treatment, this was extra torment I shouldn't have had to endure.

By the time I was in pre-op I was begging the anesthetist to knock me the hell out. Not only was I outraged, starving, and sore from the barb, I also hated being around McSteamy (he was pretty hot) while looking like Voldemort. Why couldn't this guy be homely? I was bald, had no makeup or lashes, and looked extra unattractive with my cranky face. Shame on the hospital for allowing such a dashing dude to treat me. And poor Rob. He was doing his best to be very supportive, but what could he do? Not much! However, I did give him strict instructions to greet me with some post-surgery Diet Coke and french fries. And after stewing all day because my surgery was delayed, do you know what I did when they wheeled me into the operating room? I burst into tears. Can you say basket case?!

After four hours, I woke up in the recovery room to Dr. Sarantos telling me how things went. And, once again, Rob provided me with French fries and Diet Coke upon my return from Lala Land. After all of my griping about starvation, I only ate one fry before refusing the rest. The end result of my surgery was exceptional. My still-cancerous tumor was removed, as well as two (still cancerous) lymph nodes. In an effort to make sure he had gotten everything, Dr. Sarantos also took nine more lymph nodes, which all tested negative. Cancer hadn't spread beyond where I first found it, and I got to keep a whole bunch of the "upper tier" lymph nodes. My incisions were precise, and the scars were pretty minimal. My armpit area and tricep sustained nerve damage, which has resulted in chronic numbness, but overall, surgery was a victory.

The recovery room nurses encouraged me to get up and leave fairly quickly after I woke, but I told them they were out of their minds. I wasn't going anywhere. I was extremely nauseous and felt like the room was spinning. They allowed me to go back to sleep for about an hour or so, but then they woke me up again and nudged me to go home. They also insisted I take a Percocet before I left. I should have refused it completely since Percocet makes me sick, but instead, I agreed to take half of one pill. I paid the price for my choice. When they finally got me dressed and into a wheelchair, my stomach flipped. It took me a moment to get the hospital aide to stop wheeling me forward, but once he did, I leaped out of the chair and ran across the recovery room to throw up into a garbage can. Since I had no actual food in my stomach, I just went through all of the fun heaving motions and made the awesome sounds that a vomiting person would make. I threw up nothing but air, and that experience lasted for about 10 solid minutes. I was feeling sick (obviously), slightly embarrassed from making all of those weird sounds (who wouldn't?), and exasperated that I was worse off than I should have been because of the delays. When I was done, I was wheeled out and helped into the car. On our way home, Rob stopped at a pharmacy to fill my Percocet prescription. If I was functioning properly, I would have told him not to bother. That bottle was never opened, and the contents were soon discarded.

Another fun outcome from surgery is that I left the hospital with a drain. It was a super long tube that was placed deep inside my breast, so any extra fluid would come out instead of staying inside of me, causing problems. This long drain was sewn under my left armpit to keep it in place. The rest dangled at least two feet below, outside of my body, and ended with a squeezy ball that would collect the nasty goo. I hate to get technical with y'all, but it was pretty disgusting. I couldn't even look at it for a few days and poor Rob was stuck emptying it. I was told that I had to keep the drain until my body expelled less than 30 cc's of nasty goo within a 24-hour period. I eventually ended up dealing with the drain myself, and it came out two

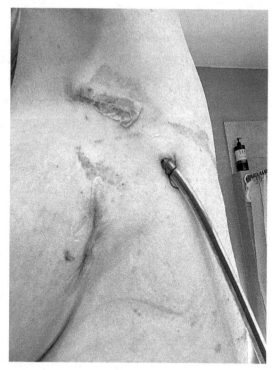

The scene after my surgery. I did not enjoy that drain.

weeks after my surgery. It was both gross and inconvenient. The long tube kept getting caught on things like chair arms and door handles, and the semi-frequent yanking on my drain made me pretty sore. I was elated when it was finally removed. Even though I did not enjoy the whole surgery experience, I was grateful not to have gone through the burdens associated with a full mastectomy. That's a far more invasive surgery, which often leads to more surgeries for reconstruction. Statistically, there were zero benefits to me having a full mastectomy, which is why I decided not to have one. Remember: all breast cancer cases are different. If you or your friends face this menace, do not compare my diagnosis or decisions with your own.

Fitzness Log

The first part of the month was a vicious test of my will to survive, but the last week came with a few bright spots. The summer sun was scorching hot and my neighborhood pool was reasonably warm, so I started venturing into it for stretching. That's all. I'd just stand in the shallow end and bend my body any way it would go. It felt great to move and the water protected me from overheating. As my go-to during previous injuries and pregnancies, I would always retreat to the water as an exercise safe haven. It provides the perfect opportunity to get fit without impact or heat becoming an issue. It's also a phenomenal place to attain elite fitness. As gentle as the water can be, swimming can be a wicked workout. I just wasn't there yet.

I also started taking Piper on tiny quarter-mile walks each day, which was great for both of us. However, one of the things I could not do was get up the very steep hill I live on. It has a 10% incline and is also known as "Killer Hill." I could make it up the less-steep roads behind my house, but not my own. One evening Rob actually drove down to pick us up because I had gotten to the bottom, but was too weak to climb back up. Propelling myself up the hill was something I was looking forward to, but that was still a while away.

Chapter 8

Radiation Equals Superpowers, Right?

August 3. Saturday.

Squeal! Alfalfa arrived. Alfalfa was the most glorious and exciting hair that ever existed. He sprouted up on the top of my head, about half an inch high, and brightened my whole world. Yes. I'm talking about a strand of hair that I named Alfalfa. At this point, I basically had no other hair at all, but out of the blue this blonde champion was there. Woohoo! I was so proud to cruise around town with one fabulous hair atop my head. The simple fact that I had any hair was a reason to celebrate. And then a week or so later, Lolita made her arrival. While Alfalfa had been stealing the show, Lolita took the lead in grand fashion. She was at least one entire inch long, and Ginger noticed her jetting out of the back of my head like the teeniest ponytail on earth. She was bold, brave, and beautiful. While many people suggested I cut Alfalfa and Lolita in efforts to keep things even, I decided to leave them be and use them as role models for my other hairs instead. If Lolita could grow one inch in one night, certainly the others could too! The leaders of my pack would be rewarded with affection, loving words, and conditioner. They would sit as a beacon of hope for all hairs to come. Great things were possible if they would just hurry up and grow.

August 12. Monday.

Chemo #8. After a fairly reasonable experience with Perjeta, I arrived to see Dr. Gordan with high hopes that things would continue to get easier. It was then that he told me that another drug called Kadcyla had just been approved for my particular situation and that he felt it was a better choice for me. It was explained to me as a sharp shooter that would seek out and kill any cancer cells floating around in my body. I would need 14 entire rounds of it. What the hell? I followed his guidance and was grateful he was staying on top of the latest research, but I was down in the dumps about tacking seven more chemo rounds to my calendar. Dr. Gordan told me that most women receiving this drug did not experience any sort of awful side effects, but I would end up as the unlucky one who did. The aftermath made me nickname this drug Godzilla.

August 13. Tuesday.

I woke up, shot out of bed, and ran into the bathroom. Facedown over our fancy toilet bowl, I heaved and heaved, but nothing came out. I also made that big baaaahhh sound that a goat makes. Strange. I didn't necessarily want to throw up, but all of the heaving alone seemed entirely pointless. I returned to bed when my body calmed down and then bolted back for more heaving. It was very odd. Apparently one of the major side effects of Kadcyla for Fitz Koehler was pointless heaving. In fact, I would spend the next few months of my life randomly heaving several times a day and in all sorts of places, while going "baaaahh" like a goat. Walking my dog and heaving – I did that a ton. Laundry and heaving – why not? Driving and heaving – thankfully only once. The mean chemo was over, but Godzilla proved to be a pain in my ass too. And since my tummy was super freaked out, my ability to eat remained limited. Sure, my taste buds were fully functional again, but Godzilla made me averse to almost everything except for the following four food items:

1. Tangerines – Six to 10 a day
2. Kind Bars – One to three a day
3. Guacamole – Too much. I'm surprised I'm not green
4. Lucky Charms with almond milk – They're magically delicious, and my body didn't reject them.

I have zero explanation as to why my body chose those items, but they were responsible for about 80% of my daily caloric intake for a very long time. I tried to squeeze in a few other options here and there, but nothing felt as easy as these four foods. And really, I needed things to be easy. I needed guarantees that I wouldn't feel crappier than I already did. As a result, I started losing weight. Weight that I did not want to lose. While the concept of weight loss usually seems exciting to most, it sucks when you're losing hard curvy muscles that you've worked tirelessly to earn. My three mini-goals were trashed. When I started this insanity, I weighed around 124 pounds. I am five foot, five and a half inches tall (yes, that half-inch matters). Within a few months, I was 115 pounds, and I was not happy. I tried to slam on the brakes of weight loss by buying some protein powder and mixing it with chocolate milk for drinking throughout the day, but that wasn't enough. My weight just kept dropping. Fortunately, I was able to stop the drop at 112. I can't imagine how sickly I'd look and feel if I had lost much more.

Now, as a fitness professional and lover of healthy bodies, I have massive respect for muscles. An understanding and appreciation that goes far beyond how they make a person look. So, let's review some of the things that happened when 12 pounds of my magnificent muscles went away:

My sleep suffered. I'm a side-sleeper who simply cannot conk out on my back. Because I lost much of my shoulder and back muscles, I ended up with throbbing pain that kept me awake, tossing and turning all night, without the ability to get comfortable. My shoulders and traps were screaming because they could no longer bear the weight of my body. This made nights miserable and my days zombie-like. And it inspired my world class physical therapist, Rob Middaugh, to continuously jam his evil thumbs into my armpit area to try and release my chest muscles. The only solution for this was more time in the gym, strengthening my back, lats, and shoulder muscles. I was actually grateful for the training assignments because at least that would be under my control. I couldn't stop the heaving, but I could definitely do whatever work it would take to regain strength and reduce pain.

My spinal discs also freaked out. Because my low back muscles were atrophied, I occasionally ended up with debilitating pain from an angry and inflamed L5 disc. When we stand for a long time gravity compresses the discs between our vertebrae. If we are strong like full-force Fitz Koehler was, our low back strength will decrease the pressure, and our discs will remain happy. But, when we don't have strong muscular structural support, pressure increases on those discs, and they often become inflamed. This happened to me twice. Once during the Monterey Bay Half Marathon weekend in November and once in February during a running conference in Vegas. If you've never experienced disc-induced pain, I'll explain. Every time I took a step with that swollen L5 disc pressing on my nerves, it knocked the wind out of me. Literally, each step stole my breath. What started out as a mildly achy back quickly became unbearable. I'd end up walking through airports slightly bent over like a woman twice my age, grimacing and crying. By the time I'd returned home from those trips, things had become so bad that I ended up crawling from my bed to my bathroom. Once again, all this while receiving zillions of messages telling me how awesome it was to see me crushing cancer so easily. Oh, the irony! The solution for me was rest, physical therapy, direct efforts to unload my spine, and a crap ton of steroids. Steroids are my friends.

My appearance suffered. It's true. While many people think that being thin is great at any cost, it's really not. I lost my curves and nothing fit. Even my running tights were loose. While I will always hold my head up high because that is who I am, I definitely struggled with this new body of mine. It's disconcerting when you put on an old favorite and it hangs like a potato sack. In fact, when packing my clothes for the Monterey Bay Half Marathon, I decided to wear a pair of dress pants and a pretty top because none of my dresses fit properly. It was a bummer because I prefer wearing dresses to these events, but I went with the only items I had that looked halfway decent. When I arrived, thinking I was going to pull it off, a friend came up to me and said, "You normally wear dresses to our parties. Are you wearing pants because your dresses are too big now?"

I was shocked. But definitely not offended. I was actually impressed by this person's accurate assessment of the situation. Even though I knew that I'd become thinner, I figured nobody else knew. Apparently, I wasn't fooling anyone. I especially wasn't fooling my mom, who one day told me that I looked like I had been through the Holocaust. Thanks, mom! She meant well in her own weird way. And, to be honest, there were quite a few times when I'd glance at my bald head and thin body and think the same thing. Where had that super fit chick with long blonde hair gone?

My face also suffered. When people lose weight, they lose it from all over, and I was no exception to that rule. Losing weight in my face left me with way more wrinkles than I'd had before this all started. I'm definitely looking forward to gaining my curvy muscles back. And, hopefully, some face fat too. For the record, I was also still hoping my nostril hair would return soon rather than later. My chronically runny nose was getting old.

August 22. Thursday.

It was finally time to get things started with Dr. Cherylle Hayes, my radiology oncologist. And I was delighted to do so since I really liked her and she was renowned as a badass cancer-killer. At my first appointment she explained some things about my particular type of breast cancer and what her thoughts were for radiation. She told me there would be 28 rounds of zapping my entire breast and lymph node area and then an extra five rounds just for the lymph nodes. I would go every weekday for 33 days. Most appointments would last 20 to 30 minutes and require absolutely no poking. Woohoo! The big thing I was concerned about was burning skin, which is often a side effect of constant radiation. I warn you, do not Google it. I shouldn't have. Many people experience such severe burns that they look like they had barbecued their boobs. No bueno. I also had some friends being treated for breast cancer whose skin was so burnt that it blistered. They couldn't even wear bras for weeks. Ouch! In order to prevent burning, I was instructed to smear Aquaphor on my skin several times a day. If I did start to experience skin irritation, I should then switch to applying Calendula cream instead and regularly place washcloths soaked in Domeboro burn solution on my breast and pits. Easy enough. I was scheduled to begin radiation on August 29th.

It had been almost two months since my last mean chemo. I was getting some energy back and was so happy to be doing even the simplest things. Taking my kids to the mall to do some school shopping felt like a win because I hadn't been able to do so since my diagnosis. It meant a lot to me to roam around the mall and purchase clothing for them. It helped me feel more like their mom again and I loved that. My taste buds were also back, so I was able to eat some things I hadn't touched in months. Going to the grocery store, picking the kids up from school, and walking the dog were other great triumphs.

August 29. Thursday.

After having a CAT scan (a series of x-rays that allows doctors to see cross-sectional images of organs, bones, and other tissues) of my chest, Dr. Hayes and her physicists mapped out a plan for my treatment. Then I showed up for radiation and the process was remarkably easy. Although I cried from nerves on the first day, they would be the last tears I would shed over radiation. Appointments were always quick, easy, and painless. Frequently, I even had a good time. If I was scheduled at 9 a.m., I'd traditionally get sent into the women's changing area to put on a gown about five minutes prior. During my first visit, I was told that the blue gowns stacked on the bench were average size, while the yellow gowns were extra large. *Hmmm. Those yellow gowns could be fun.* Nonetheless, I'd toss on a gown, throw my belongings into a locker, and then go into the big radiation room to be zapped.

My radiation techs Morgan, Kayleigh, and Scott, would have me lie on a skinny table with my head on a pillow that was specifically molded for my noggin. Once there, I would have to slide my arms out of my gown and fold it down, so my chest was exposed. Then, I'd reach my arms up over my head and grab onto handles that jetted out of the table behind me. As soon as I was in that position, the techs would line up the zapper precisely to match the Sharpie Xs that were drawn onto my left breast. As soon as I was lined up, my techs would leave the room, and the massive machine would start doing loops around me. Every day I'd first get a CAT scan to make sure my body was in the proper position, and then I'd get zapped. The whole process took no more than 10 to 15 minutes, and absolutely nothing about it hurt. The only thing that ever did cause irritation was the nonsense stuff like dealing with an itchy nose or a wedgie once I was told to remain perfectly still.

I can honestly say that I enjoyed this part of my treatment. I was feeling a bit more like myself, and my techs were great people to be around. They dealt with so many somber situations that I think they appreciated the energy I brought in each day. We'd chat about Gator sports, fitness, my races, and more while they were setting things up. And they'd play country music for me while I was being zapped. Eventually, I got sick of the blue gowns and switched to the monstrous, but pretty, yellow gowns. I decided they were a lot more fun, so I chose to wear them regularly, and everyone would have a good laugh. The other thing I liked about radiation was the fresh-baked cookies. Apparently these folks knew how to

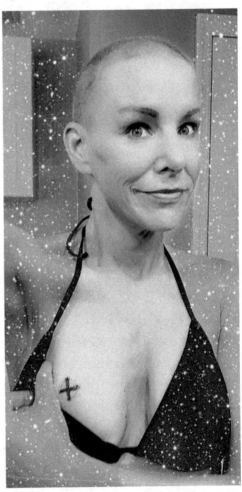

X marks the spot for radiation.

181

cook more than just people. Several times a day, they'd bake batches of Otis Spunkmeyer cookies and leave them individually wrapped in the lobby. I almost always treated myself to one before I left. Chocolate chip, of course. I quickly dubbed them radiation cookies and I'll tell you what: radiation cookies are delicious!

I was secretly hoping that superpowers would be a fun side effect of my radiation. Many of our favorite superheroes and supervillains were blessed with extraordinary abilities after interacting with radioactive substances. Spiderman, for example, gained his powers after being bitten by a radioactive spider. The Fantastic Four got their fancy powers zooming in a spaceship through a cloud of cosmic radiation. The Hulk gained his strength after he was exposed to gamma radiation. You get the picture. I was really looking forward to flying, shooting lasers from my eyes, or making supersonic sounds. #RadiationPerks

Besides my daily zaps, I'd go in to see Dr. Hayes every Wednesday. Since I never showed up in crisis, our visits were kind of airy, and we often chatted about things other than cancer. In fact, at the beginning of my treatment she encouraged me to do a special hip-hop fitness class with her. I wasn't necessarily feeling my best, but I got caught up in the moment and quickly agreed to meet her at our gym for it. Rob and I joked that we should show up wearing tracksuits, gold chains, and bucket hats à la Run DMC. However, we chose to wear regular workout clothes instead. The class was packed, and the two of us hung out in the back of the room trying not to garner attention. Our moves were half funky and half dorky, but we had a lot of fun and laughed a lot.

Back to radiation. Along the way, my skin ended up looking like I had a mild sunburn. Thankfully I didn't experience the severe burning many of my friends did. If I had to pinpoint the worst side effect of radiation during my treatment, I'd choose relentless itchiness. Dr. Hayes told me not to scratch because it would make things worse, and I tried really hard not to, but it was a pest. Fellow cancer patients have asked me for suggestions to avoid radiation burns. And I think that having young, healthy skin goes a long way. Of course, you can't control your age, but I do believe that being younger was a real advantage here. I met a bunch of older women in the changing room who showed me their burned and blistered breasts. I felt for them. Maybe the universe gave me a break with radiation because I was so crazy sick from chemo? Perhaps. Beyond having young, healthy skin, I was religious about using the Aquaphor, Calendula, and Domeboro as directed.

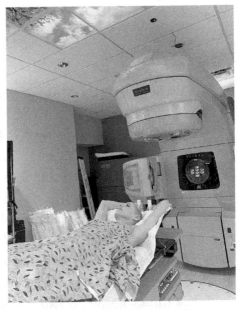

Ready to get zapped with radiation.

Many people complain about having to go to radiation every single weekday. And I was warned in advance that it might be tiring. I bet it is for people who have to drive really far to get there. I can certainly understand how a long commute would've been draining. I also think it'd be pretty rough if I were going through the mean chemo at the same time. But for my personal situation, living just a 10-minute drive from The Cancer Center, I really didn't mind it at all. In fact, my daily appointments kind of kicked off a little bit of a routine for me. I would head to radiation every morning around 9 a.m., and then I'd go to the gym for some strength training and stretching. Since I wasn't crazy sick anymore, I appreciated getting back to having a routine and some semblance of normalcy. The weeks when I had chemo and radiation were tougher than others, but I look back at radiation as a reasonably happy experience.

My exciting new schedule:

- 9 a.m. Radiation
- 10 a.m. Gym
- 11 a.m. Physical Therapy
- 12 p.m. Lunch

- 12:30 p.m. Nap time!
- 2:45 p.m. Pick up Kids from School

Fitzness Log

August was a pretty exciting month for me because, after a three-month hiatus, I finally returned to the Gainesville Health and Fitness Center. I felt like a fish being thrown back into the water. It was incredibly refreshing and a HUGE milestone for me. Sure, I wasn't as strong as I was the last time I was there, but I was pumped to start making progress again. In fact, that was something I really looked forward to. Pre-cancer, my workouts were on cruise control. I wasn't chasing any athletic or aesthetic goals, despite putting in a lot of hard work. But now I was working with a definable mission: I wanted to, at a minimum, be able to lift as much, run as much, and be as flexible as I was before.

I took things slowly for two reasons. First, I didn't want to do harm. Surgery and chemo had weakened me and I knew I was susceptible to injury if I pushed the envelope. Second, my body was only capable of going slow. My time in the gym was dedicated to strength training using free weights, machines, bands, cables, and kettlebells. I also focused on stretching. Cardio was reserved for walking Piper, who deserved as much of it as I could give her. For my legs, I did my Strength Training for Runners Workout (available on Fitzness.com). That included lunges, squats, lateral gait with bands, chicken wings, straddle lifts, and hamstring curls. Since I was still recovering from surgery, my upper body workouts were limited. I mostly focused on getting range of motion back in my left shoulder. And I visited my physical therapist for pain relief twice a week. My return to the gym was something I'd been pining for, so getting there felt like a major conquest. Point awarded to ... Fitz Koehler!

As for walking up killer hill, I was only making the climb if Rob was behind me with his hand on my back pushing. When I'd fatigue, I'd whine, "Push harder!" and we'd laugh about my wimpiness.

Chapter 9

The Bright Side of Poop on My Face

September 5. Thursday.

Sometimes I'm a foolish person. Remember when I told you that stubbornness was both my greatest asset and my greatest curse? This is a prime example of when it was a curse. I was scheduled for an MRI at 12:15 p.m. to take another peek at the lesion that was seen on my right breast at the start. You know, the one that the radiologist deemed non-threatening. They were also going to look at the rest of my chest and organs to make sure cancer hadn't popped up anywhere else. Now, considering the way my first MRI went, the original game plan was for me to take some sort of anti-anxiety medication before I tried that again. However, Ginger was scheduled to cheer at her high school's football game that night, and I didn't want to be loopy. So, instead of taking the single pill that could have saved me from torture, I moronically chose to bypass it and suck it up emotionally. That was a big fail.

The second I entered the MRI room, I started panicking, hyperventilating and crying. It was basically a replay of the nightmare I had at the start of this saga, which costarred the same cranky MRI lady. Why I did that to myself, I will never know. But if I am ever scheduled for another

MRI, I will likely require crack cocaine to get me through it. I jest, but come on! It was a dumb move. As you can imagine, the MRI lady was as happy to see me as I was to see her. But I did get through it, and the results were perfect. They didn't see any cancer anywhere. Half a point awarded to ... Fitz Koehler! Note: I took away half a point for being a dumbass.

September 11. Wednesday.

This was an exhilarating day for ~~Voldermort~~ me! For two months, I had been dealing with the frustrations of having no lashes. I can understand how many of you are thinking, "Come on, Fitz. They're just eyelashes. It's no biggie." But the reality is, without lashes defining part of my face, I looked undeniably weird. I would try to compensate for the loss with eyeliner, but it never worked out as I'd hoped. I even went through a bunch of Youtube tutorials created by beauty gurus who lost their lashes due to chemo or Alopecia. They were slightly helpful, and I did my best to follow the good advice, but nothing ever really made up for my eye-nudity. I basically just had to ride things out until my natural lashes started to regrow. And eventually, they did.

I'm going to backtrack a bit here. While I've always been a pretty natural girl when it comes to style and makeup, that doesn't mean I haven't put some sort of effort into my appearance. Obviously, I've put in effort on my physique through exercise and eating wisely, but I have also done some basic things to look prettier. One thing I do before I step on a stage or go on television is to get a spray tan. My glorious Irish ancestry has yielded ghostly white skin, and I combat that with a little help from a fantastic little Gainesville salon called LAE Beauty. For over a decade, I've made a spray tan at LAE a must-do before getting on a plane or going in front of a camera. Both my father and maternal grandmother died of skin cancer, so it's nice to be able to get a little color on my skin without the fear of dying from it. Sometimes I choose the Mystic Tanning Booth, in which I'm sprayed automatically and privately. Other times I choose a custom airbrush tan, which is done in a little room where I stand in my thong undies and get sprayed by one of the LAE staffers.

While I'm generally not an exhibitionist, I can get past my own shyness and disrobe because these women are professionals who probably couldn't care less about my nudity. Their reactions during my continuously drastic physical changes were very professional too. Not once did any of them mention my weight loss or my skinhead situation. They also never commented on my post-surgery scars, which they would get an eyeful of. I never felt judged or embarrassed about my ever-changing appearance and that speaks volumes about the kindness and professionalism of the lovely ladies of LAE. We did, however, have a bunch of laughs when they coated my bald head with the tanning spray. I mean, what were we supposed to do? Leave it super pale on top of my bronze body? That would have looked strange. So, yeah. We sprayed my naked noggin. It was awesome.

LAE is also where I got my lash extensions done. I remember back to the start of my treatments when I told the owner Kelley how badly I was hoping not to lose my lashes. She was quick to assure me that as long as I had nubs for lashes, she could attach extensions. I hung on that promise when my lashes fell out. So much so that I looked at my super zoom mirror every day after to see if any tiny lashes had appeared. Eventually, along with Lolita and Alfalfa, they did. Right before my first race back, teeny tiny baby lashes made their way back onto my face. I was thrilled to be able to take my lash nubs back to LAE so that they could make my eyes look fabulous again. It sounds like a small thing, but it felt like a major achievement to get something back again. After all of the setbacks and losses I'd suffered, I was finally making gains. Not only did I leave LAE with beautiful lashes that day, but Kelley refused to let me pay for them. It meant as much to her to give me lashes as it did for me to receive them. How lucky am I? Point awarded to … Fitz Koehler!

September 8. Sunday.

Perspective is everything. Isn't it? It's been a critical tool throughout my entire life, but during my breast cancer treatment, it was more valuable than diamonds. It gifted me with the ability to chronically look on the bright side, and on this day, that skill came in handy. Big time. I was walking Piper around my neighborhood and had just waved at my friend Beth who was out in her garage. Beth had also had a difficult year. Her young husband passed away in early May. We briefly connected in July with a big hug and a short conversation that didn't need to be had. Both of our lives had been turned upside down, in very different ways, and there was nothing anyone could do to rescue either of us from our predicaments. We just had to keep trudging along until things got better. While other people were trying to magically solve our problems, we didn't do that to or for each other. When we'd cross paths, we would just smile and give each other a knowing nod.

Back to my walk with Piper. I had just passed Beth's house when BAM! I was hit in the face by something hard. I stopped, squealed, and grabbed my face. I was standing in the middle of the road in disbelief when Beth came running over to see if I was okay. "Beth," I asked. "Is there poop on my face?" "Yes!" she replied. We stared at each other in disbelief and a few moments later proceeded to die laughing. We were buckled over in hysterics. I don't think either of us had laughed that hard in months. Sure, standing there with dung all over my forehead, nose, and chin was utterly grotesque. But quite frankly, I couldn't have been more thankful to the ridiculous bird who dropped the big doo-doo on my mug. Beth and I both needed that laugh. Once we recovered from our sides splitting, she offered to go get me some paper towels. I was happy to take her up on her offer. And from that day on, whenever we see each other, and one of us asks "How are you?" the other enthusiastically replies, "I've got no poop on my face!" And that's the perspective you gain when you know that things could always be worse.

September 14. Saturday.

After a long 2-month break, I was finally getting back on an airplane for Eva's *Women Run the D* Half Marathon and 5K in Detroit. The time off from travel had been beneficial. It allowed me to recover properly from surgery, get much of the mean chemo out of my system, and more. I wasn't 100%, but I was a zillion times better than I had been the last time I stepped on a stage in Denver. I had about a centimeter's worth of little dirty blond hairs all over my head, and I was excited to show them off. Sure, the color was a little weird for me, and the hair was a bit patchy, but I didn't care. Things were looking up. It was also great that my first race back was in Michigan. I have so many close friends there, including Eva's Epic Races team. I've been announcing this event since 2014 and it's always felt like home.

Cruising through the Atlanta airport was a real kick. I had so many flashbacks to my tribulations in that airport. Memories of my panicked searches for decent food and decent bathrooms struck me, as well as reminders of the time I got off of my flight from Gainesville and realized that my vision had suddenly gone entirely wonky. My eyes have always been sharp, and I've never worn glasses, so you can imagine my shock when I walked off the jetway, and everything was blurry. I could barely read the gate signs to find out which plane I should board. Things stayed super blurry for a very long time, and my eyes still haven't returned to normal. Much like losing my nostril hair, no one ever told me that chemo could screw with my eyesight. Besides reminiscing, I was giddy to be back on the road and back to my races.

September 15. Sunday.

I simply cannot find the words to express to you what a joy it is to wake up knowing what lies ahead for me on race days. Even though a long break was definitely in order, two months was far too long for me to be off the microphone. I was chomping at the bit to get over to Belle Isle and get going with all of our athletes. As I left my hotel, a friend asked me to get her some tampons. The front desk lady gave me a handful, and I laughed as I shoved them into my bag, knowing I'd never have to be the girl stranded without feminine products again. Since my cancer is hormonal, my chemo and follow-up drugs would put me into early menopause, which meant I wouldn't have to have any more periods. Hooray for me! Apparently, there were a few perks to all of this nonsense after all. None were worth the cost, but I've decided to find the bright spots where they exist. And for those gals reading this and wondering what that's like – I've had no menopause-style symptoms at all. As things are right now, it looks like I'm getting a free pass on that. Perhaps I won't have to deal with the crappy stuff menopause brings at all.

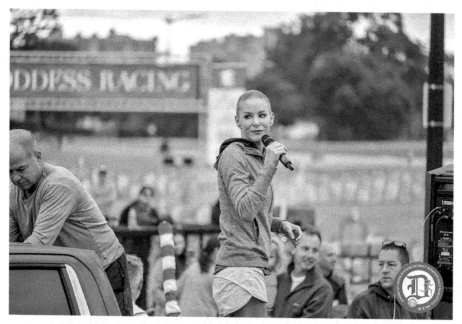

Thrilled to be back on the microphone for Women Run the D.
Photo by Greg Sadler

Pre-race, endless amounts of my Michigan friends stopped by for hugs, short bits of chit chat, and plenty of oohs and ahhs over my stubbly head. My Hotties made a huge showing, and I loved getting to fawn all over them. It's such a gift when I get to witness the people I've guided through major weight loss, strength gains, and race prep do their thing. It's a very similar kind of pride and joy that comes along with being a parent. My Hotties, my runners, my Fitzness folks – in general – are always telling me how much I mean to them and how much they appreciate my guidance. It fills my heart up to the brim and certainly makes me feel like I've chosen the right career path.

Before we kicked things off, I spent some time recognizing our Epic Heart Heroes. They are women who have overcome significant issues with their tickers, and I tell you, their stories are moving. We've had plenty of Heart Heroes over the years who've had transplants, bypass surgeries and more, and now they're out living life to the fullest. Not only do I enjoy giving them the recognition they deserve for being courageous, but I also enjoy seeing other runners learn from their experiences. Too many of our Heart Heroes had symptoms that they ignored for almost too long. They tell similar tales of feeling tired or breathless for a while and just thinking they were being wimpy. Some thought they could sleep off flu-like symptoms. Over the years, many of them have shared how they accidentally discovered they were on the brink of death. It's quite concerning how many people ignore symptoms. For most folks, nausea and breathlessness are not normal. Those experiences usually occur when our body is in crisis and trying to tell us that something is wrong. If you have bizarre feelings that are brief and mild, that's fine. But if you have issues that refuse to go away, get worse, or come on quick and sharp – go to a damn doctor! Too many stubborn mules are found dead on the floor or end up with Stage 4 nightmares because they failed to act on their own behalf. Don't be that mule.

Back to the race. I summarized the Heart Hero stories, but tried to do so in a way that would resonate with the rest of our athletes. I hope they'll get proper medical attention if they're ever in a similar boat. Heart disease is the top killer of American women, and a huge percentage of those deaths are preventable. I took the opportunity to throw in a plug for mammograms and self-exams while I was at it, using my stubbly head as a quality reminder.

Our crowd of mostly female athletes was boisterous at the start line, and the majority of them celebrated their finishes with big joy as well. Our course was changed up a bit due to flooding on Belle Isle and our finish line chute wrapped around a beautiful and large fountain, with my stage right at the finish. It was a pretty lovely alternative to our regular course, and I hope Eva decides to keep it. It drizzled all morning, but no one seemed to mind. Our spectators were properly rambunctious, and one of them came dressed in a taco costume with a dachshund dressed as a hotdog. They danced enthusiastically for hours and kept me and everyone else giggling all morning. It was yet another reason I love the running community. Some people will do just about anything to make the experience more fun.

Meanwhile my Hottie, Valerie Diem, kept me cozy and fed. She is an Epic Heart Hero who's also a stroke victim. She works hard to stay fit, has a sarcastic wit, and is always a delight to hang out with. When she finished the 5K, she brought me a cooler full of snacks and drinks, an umbrella, a blanket, and some other niceties. She and my other Hotties gathered around my stage when they were done running in support of the other athletes and me. How cool is that? Throughout this lengthy experience my mother has been very concerned about me traveling while sick. What mother wouldn't be? However, I have always been able to assure her of two things that I think are pretty impressive. First, at every single race I work, there is always an ambulance or medical team nearby. So, if I ever went downhill while announcing, I was in the perfect place for it to be addressed. Who else has that kind of proximity to medical care on the job? Not many. Second, the running community has kept an incredibly keen eye out for me all year. It's as though I've had thousands of caretakers all around the country willing to do anything to keep me well. While it is truly my job to take care of them, this year my athletes turned the tables on me, and it's been very appreciated.

The other person whom I treasure time with is Greg Sadler, a long-time Epic Races professional photographer and good friend of mine. Greg and I met during my first race for Eva, and he instantly declared me his favorite subject to shoot. It's an excellent deal because he's provided me with tons of beautiful announcing pictures. In reality, he works with a ton of gorgeous individuals. I'm sure I'm not at the top of that list, but he has captured many incredible moments of me with my athletes. Whether I'm on my stage yelling "GO," escorting athletes across their finish lines, or sashaying around the course with my big-arse cowbell. I'm probably like his Queen of Candids. He's also a bit of a renaissance man, which makes our conversations incredible. We can talk about parenting, politics, sports, education, travel, science, and more, all within a tiny window of time.

The next week at home was dedicated to resting, moderately exercising, another echocardiogram, and a painful goodbye with Lilly. Sadly, she was transferred from the FCS in Gainesville to one about 45 minutes south in Ocala. Oy! That was an emotional good-bye. Lilly had become a bit of a safety net during chemo, and I really appreciated her expert care and compassion. I know I didn't *need* her, but I definitely *wanted* her. She had a unique ability to make a miserable situation manageable and had truly protected me on many occasions. Of course, she rescued me from a stressful conversation on my first day, but she also shielded me from a few others. On one of my worst days, there was an overly chatty woman who liked to roam around the infusion room talking everyone's ears off. She was headed toward me when Lilly hustled over and whispered, "Close your eyes and pretend you're sleeping." I instantly snapped my eyes shut and left them that way until the threat to my peace had passed. It was a simple act, but it mattered. Lilly never screwed up a stick, and I liked her as a person. After radiation one day, I walked over to give her a little gift and thank you card. I hugged her tightly as I choked back the tears. Lilly and I still stay in touch and I hope we always do. Once Lilly left, I claimed John Colon as my permanent nurse.

September 18. Wednesday.

Hallelujah. This was the day I had been pining away for. I finally had enough hair that I could go into Kristen's salon and have it dyed platinum. After spending most of my life as a lighter blonde, the super dirty and patchy darker blonde that had grown in felt a bit sketchy. I was one million percent grateful to have a teeny little two-centimeter layer of hair all over my head, but I wanted my softer halo back. And for those of you who are horrified by the thought, this came with complete approval from Dr. Gordan. To say that I bounded into her salon that day is an understatement. Our last few appointments were heartbreaking and so symbolic of my lack of control in my life. The fact that I was going to get to choose a color for my stubble just elated me. Kristen took her time to assess what strategy would work best and then started painting my head with her products.

I was crazy excited for a fantastic outcome, but I was also slightly terrified that dying my hair blond would make my new hair fall out. I should have just trusted Kristen's expertise, but I was bottling up a bit of anxiety at the thought of returning to full bald again. I've heard horror stories from others going blonde. When my 60 minutes in her chair were up, my hair was totally platinum, and so was my smile. Yet again, I was brought to tears in her salon. But this time, they were happy tears. It felt so good to be making my comeback. Baby steps, of course, but I finally felt kind of happy with the girl I saw in the mirror again. Point awarded to ... Fitz Koehler!

My plan was to spike my hair up once it came in. And I mean way up. I decided that I wanted a faux hawk (mohawk without the sides of my head shaved). *A very tall faux hawk.* When I told Ginger, she was fairly appalled and said, "No, you're not." "Yes, I am!" I responded. We went back and forth with "You are NOT having a faux hawk!" and "Watch me!" which became very fun. I bought several types of gel and in December, I was able to form the hair I had into a point. By April, that point would be three inches high. My goal was to keep it going up until it could all fall down when parted in the center. The back and forth with Ginger continued, and it delighted me to torture her this way.

I'd like to take this time to share some advice for those of you who like to talk about chemo hair. Stop it! I can't tell you how many people enthusiastically told me, "Do you know your hair may come in completely different when it returns? It may be really curly or really dark!" Ummmm. Eff you, idiots! I know, that's harsh. But think about it. What you're really saying to that cancer patient is, "Hey! You know that hair you had, that you loved, and lost? You may never see it again!" Gosh, that's annoying. Everyone knows hair often returns a different color, an odd texture, or even with curls. No cancer patient enjoys that possibility. Of course, the folks saying it are trying to connect, but it's not a fun conversation for the patient, and we all think you're an ass for your enthusiasm. So, just stop. Talk about the weather or politics or religion instead. Trust me, those topics are far more delightful. And here's something else to consider. A few chemotherapy drugs are so toxic that some people never have their hair grow back. Never! Imagine how stressful your annoying hair comments might be to that person. Your fun conversation makes us grind our teeth, so just back off. We'll deal with our new hair however we want, if and when we're lucky enough to get it back.

September 20. Friday.

I was ecstatic to board a plane to Los Angeles. I was headed west to announce the inaugural DC Batman Run Series 5K, and I'd have my noisy sidekick Rudy by my side. It was like a sister event to our DC Wonder Woman Run Series, and we were stoked to add Batman to the mix. Like Wonder Woman, Batman is iconic, and the crowds that show up to race in LA mean business. Since I enjoy torturing Rudy so much, I declared that I would be Batman for the weekend, and he would be my Robin. I even threatened to make him wear red tights, which never actually happened. He's such a fantastic sport.

I had a surprisingly gratifying encounter during my flight from Atlanta to Los Angeles. I was seated in a row for three people and ended up chatting with the two gentlemen to my left. We were silent for the first half of our four-hour journey while I was writing this book, but soon we began chatting. The 70-ish man in the middle seat was a former university president who was on his way to give a lecture in LA, and the 40-something man in the aisle seat was a technology pro who was headed to Hawaii for vacation. And then there was me, the girl in the window seat. When it was my turn to share what I did, the two guys asked if they could guess what I did. It seemed kind of odd, but also kind of fun, so I agreed. I had confidence they would never come up with "race announcer."

Mr. Middle Seat started things off. His first guess was that I was the nanny for the wealthy family in first class. He said he knew that's what I did because he could tell the twin babies loved me during the boarding process. "Nope. I'm just really good with babies," I said. He was shocked by my response and then took another guess about me being a creative type who worked in the entertainment industry or public relations. Wrong again. I was fascinated by the process and their guesses because I knew it was my stubbly platinum hair that was stimulating their thought process. *Who was this woman with the blonde buzz cut?* After Mr. Middle Seat struck out, Mr. Aisle Seat took a few stabs. Marketing? No. Fashion Designer? Ha! No, but thank you. His guess made me feel good. This was all very amusing.

Eventually, I revealed what I actually do and then exposed the truth about my hair. That's when the good stuff squished out as Mr. Aisle Seat almost lost his mind. He divulged that what he *really believed* was that I was an edgy, artsy type on my way home to Los Angeles. And, more specifically, he thought I was a liberal protester who surely wore a vagina hat on weekends and waved vulgar signs around town. Holy cow! I laughed so hard and loved every minute of it.

The thing that I appreciated the most is that neither of them had predicted I was sick or battling cancer. Though I had felt like the walking posterboard for cancer, roaming the country bald for many months, the wee little blonde locks on my head had changed all of that. I wasn't a nanny, a marketing director, or an angry protester. But in my book, all of those things were a trillion times better than a poster child for cancer. Point awarded to ... Fitz Koehler!

September 21. Saturday.

I can't tell you how delighted I was to shimmy into my black Batman tutu and tank top. My work wardrobe simply can't be topped, and this new theme was too much fun. I headed over to City Hall for one of the most fun days of the year. I believe we had about 5,000 athletes registered, about a million spectators, and a swarm of professionals from the Warner Brothers company and DC Comics. Besides putting on a rock star nighttime 5K, we would be celebrating the 80th anniversary of Batman. We hosted the expo and bib-pickup portion of this event throughout the day before the event, so we were beyond busy. Most of our athletes showed up very early to gather their stuff and also to enjoy the festival, which was pretty darn cool. Warner Brothers brought out the Batmobile and Batman himself to do meet and greets and pose for pictures with fans. We had a giant Lego Batman set up and a ton of other Batman-themed activations. Rudy and I spent the day plugging our vendors, sharing important race info, and entertaining the crowds. Looking back, we knocked it out of the park. From beginning to end, spirits were intensely cheerful, and the excitement was palpable. While our DC Wonder Woman Run Series is visually spectacular because 90% of our athletes come dressed as Wonder Woman in some form, this Batman event was cool because the entire DC Comic Universe was represented. The great majority of folks were dressed in a Batman theme, but we also saw a ton of Jokers, Harley Quinns, Mr. Freezes, The Penguins, The Riddlers, The Scarecrows, and Batgirls. Our event tents, flags, and video graphics were gorgeous, and I reveled in being part of such a masterpiece.

Since it was a scorcher, my athletes made every effort to make sure I was healthy. Sweet Shelly Villalobos and her husband Eddie roamed around the city to get me snacks and beverages throughout the day. Others stopped by to offer me

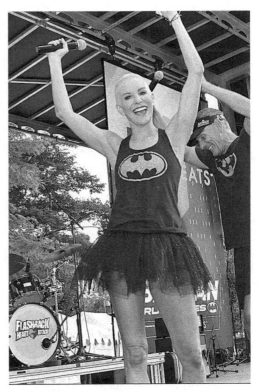

Crazy fun with Rudy at the DC Batman Run, Los Angeles. Photo by Jay Sutherland/Sport Photo Group

drinks and protein bars. My blood sugar dropped pretty low in the heat, so these gifts saved me from taking a turn for the worst.

Having Warner Brothers and DC Comics on-site made things interesting. They had invested a lot into promoting our event, they were bringing some big wigs out to take part in a declaration ceremony, and they brought a ton of employees out to run. Plus, they owned the brand. Making them happy was important. We wanted to make sure that their needs and those of our athletes were met, so we sat down for a meeting to discuss how things were going to play out. I enjoyed meeting their expectations and garnering their faith that everything else was done properly. They were the Warner Brothers and DC entertainment pros, but we were the race pros. I couldn't be happier with the way things played out.

197

About 90 minutes before the 5K began, we took to the main stage for some uproarious fun. Our participants were total gamers, which meant all of our contests had tons of entrants and endless laughter. Our Batman trivia contest was first and it inspired fascinating conversations. If they knew the answer, athletes were instructed to run to the stage and use my foot as a buzzer. I'm grateful my foot wasn't broken into a million pieces that day. Batman fans know their stuff and would sprint to the stage to be the first to whack my foot. Fortunately, they were gentle enough to cause no harm.

Next up was our magnificent costume contest. Holy cow, these people were hard-core creative! I felt like half of them could jump into a movie role and folks would believe that they were the real character. I interviewed each contestant about their attire and included questions like, "If you were to go party with a Super Friend, who would it be?" and "If you were going to battle a DC villain, who would you choose and why?" Their responses were all very clever, and the crowd engagement was staggering. They loved celebrating their fellow athletes.

Last on our list was a new segment I created called the "Talk like Batman" contest. Basically, I compiled a list of real and fake Batman quotes for contestants to read in their best Batman voice. If you don't recall, the recent movie versions of Batman – think Christian Bale – The Dark Knight speaks with a deep, gravelly voice. Watching and listening to our contestants trying to talk like that was awesome. Some quotes were legit, such as, "It's not who I am underneath, but what I do that defines me." But hearing them say things like, "Are you going to eat the rest of your French fries?" Or "Excuse me, do you know where I can find the little boys room?" was hilarious. Our spectators lost their minds!

Once we wrapped up the contests, it was quickly time to do the national anthem and go to the start line. We had a bit of commotion because a thousand or so people waited until the last minute to show up to get their gear. It wasn't a smart idea for them, but our crew ended up finding a solution. Rudy stayed on the main stage while I hurried over to the start line to launch our 5K. With the official Warner Brothers Batman by my side, I got to play ringleader for one of the most exhilarating crowds I've ever worked with. Looking back, I'm semi-surprised that we didn't all spontaneously combust. It was that raucous. With the crowd in a complete frenzy, I yelled, "Batman, set, GO!" and the happiest group of Super Friends and villains paraded by me, waving, shouting, and bursting with joy.

Once everyone crossed the start line, it was time to leap onto our finish line stage to welcome our champions. Our athletes were just as fired up at the finish line as they had been at the start because the course was jam-packed with surprises. I can't tell you all of the details, because I didn't get to actually run the race, but I can tell you that a highlight was running through a tunnel filled with purple lights and smoke, while listening to classic Batman music. I usually say that I eat runners for breakfast, but on this day, I ate them for dinner and they were a five-star gourmet meal. I legitimately feed off of the joy of my people. It's indescribable how an experience like this negated so much of the bad stuff. It certainly didn't erase all of the scary, sick, and stressful times I'd endured, but it did boost my quality of life by a million percent.

After the final athlete crossed the finish line, the party continued with our 80's cover band, "Flashback Heart Attack" performing on the main stage. Hordes of people had tons of post-race energy and were using it to dance the night away. At

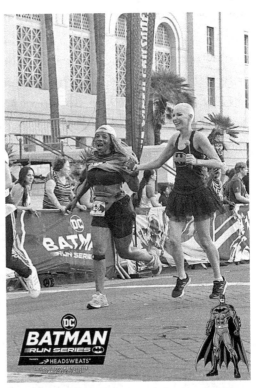

Running Vikki Richardson through the finish of the DC Batman Run, Los Angeles. Photo by Jay Sutherland/Sport Photo Group

some point, I had to interrupt the concert to do a little bit of business for Warner Brothers and DC Comics. We had a short ceremony where the City of Los Angeles declared this to be Official Batman Day, and we acknowledged a local kid who got to turn on the Bat-Signal, which shone brightly on one of the stages at Warner Brother Studios. By the time we finished that night, Rudy and I were hungry, exhausted, and completely fulfilled. When I woke up the next morning, I went straight to the airport so I could make it home in time for chemo and radiation the following day.

September 23. Monday.

The weird thing about going in for such intense medical care the day after a high-energy race weekend was always the contrast. No matter how many times I did it, I'd always walk into the cancer center scratching my head wondering how the hell I continuously boomeranged from one extreme to another. I mean, seriously? I was literally just on stage with Batman while leading the charge for thousands of raucous athletes. In what screwed up story do I go from that to chemo and radiation? Mine, I guess. It was bizarre, but if I had to be a cancer patient, I wouldn't have wanted it any other way. I felt sad for my fellow patients who didn't have so much goodness to look forward to during their battles. And while they probably didn't have the opportunity to work with The Dark Knight, I hoped they all had something special to cling to.

I felt a little mischievous that morning, so I bounced into radiation eager to tell the techs about my weekend. But first, I had to use restraint when I entered the changing room. There was a cord that stuck out of the wall with the words "Call for Help" above it. I had looked at this cord about 18 times already and was always curious about who would come if I pulled it. Would an alarm sound? Would some sort of message be played over the intercom? Would the radiation techs, administrative employees, or doctors come running? I desperately wanted to know. However, to avoid unnecessary chaos, I restrained myself. Instead, I settled for posing with the cord and taking a smirking selfie with a Snapchat filter, which put devil horns on my head. If I could go back in time, I might actually pull it. Even though I was in a serious medical facility, shenanigans are a fantastic part of life.

After a lovely chat and some zapping from my techs, I headed over to receive chemo. I mentioned this earlier, but one of the protocols that comes with some drugs is a strictly timed observation period after they are delivered. For example, Godzilla was to be dripped into me through the IV over a 30-minute time frame, which was precisely controlled by the computer on my IV pole. Once the bag of Godzilla was empty, my nurse John observed me for another 30 minutes to make sure I didn't have any foul reactions to the drug. But since I'm a squirmy girl and wasn't worried about allergic reactions, I made all sorts of efforts to get out of chemo jail. Usually, this came by way of me telling John that he wasn't observing me properly. He'd be tending to his other patients or documenting stuff on his computer and I expected to be fully, and properly, observed. When I'd eventually become a pain in the ass, he would respond by crouching down behind some object while peeking around the corner of it to stare at me with big bugged eyes. It was so funny. Chemo might have started out as an intensely stressful experience, but my visits were becoming lighter, and I really appreciated the levity. Still, the combination of a busy travel weekend, Benadryl, chemo, and radiation kicked my booty, so off to crash at home with sweet Piper I went.

Fitzness Log

I'd been making real progress with the range of motion in my left shoulder and was continuing to hit the gym for strength training a few times a week. It was *interesting* to be in a fitness center and be less-than. Less than what? Less than the previous version of Fitz Koehler. That girl was an absolute beast. This girl had to sit down and rest after doing 10 lunges. This girl had to take an extra-long break between sets of military press using dumbbells. I used the word "interesting" because I didn't feel bad about it. Instead, I thought about all of the people who never even attempt to exercise for fear of not living up to arbitrary expectations. It's okay to start behind where you once were. It's okay to make gradual gains in capabilities. The only thing that ever matters is that you're showing up and moving forward. Again, I was ecstatic to have a challenge laid out in front of me and to be making minor improvements. It's the argument I've made to my clients for decades when they've worried about feeling inadequate while exercising. Zero people in the gym surrounding me knew that I was doing less than I used to. Nobody was judging me. Nobody cared. Was I on the weaker side? Definitely! Was I moving toward the stronger side? Hell yes. Should it matter to anyone on the planet other than myself? The answer to that question is a resounding "no."

My walks with Piper became longer, and I was able to conquer killer hill on my own. It was another milestone. Double points awarded to … Fitz Koehler! And triple points awarded to … Rob Koehler! (Because he didn't have to push me up killer hill anymore.)

Chapter 10

The Thing With Pink Ribbons ...

October 1. Tuesday.

The beginning of Breast Cancer Awareness Month had arrived and, for me, it was going to be tricky. Obviously I was and am grateful for all of the love, care, and action that society has poured into curing this evil beast. I've benefited so much from it, and so have many of my friends. With the intentions to raise funds, awareness, and encourage people to do regular breast exams, it's an extraordinary thing. However, I was daunted by the fact that I'll never be able to just forget about my horrible experience with breast cancer. It seemed like the entire country had decked itself out in pink everything. FCS and the hospital next door had staked about 492 million flamingos into the grounds of the property. It was absolutely adorable, but it also made me cringe. I hate breast cancer. In fact, I hate all cancer.

For the record, I think it's tacky when people toss around the word hate. Hate comes with an awful lot of negative energy, and I'm just not willing to contaminate myself with it. Do you really hate pickles? Do you truly hate that politician? It's a strong word, and I've spent my life reserving real hatred for only the worst things: terrorism and cancer. But yeah, I definitely do hate cancer. And I finally figured out why I don't wear the ribbons. It's because they make me feel like a victim, and I don't think this nasty disease deserves a place of honor on my chest. Make sense? I'm not rejecting the goodwill. I'm rejecting cancer. It's probably an idiotic protest, but I've sought out control where I can get it. Perhaps I will change my mind about it someday.

October 3. Thursday.

I was 15 weeks out from my final round of mean chemo and had finally grown a full head of stubby hair. To clarify, it was still just half-inch long, but it was thick again, and there weren't any more bald spots. People would comment on how quickly they thought my hair was returning. In reality, it was behind the curve, but that was okay. I was grateful for what I had. If you look it up, statistics suggest most people grow about a half-inch of head hair per month. Mine had grown about half an inch in almost four months. It's not a complaint, it was just my reality. And I knew this because Parker and I would regularly measure my hair. Sure, it was a silly thing to do, but I was curious, and we continuously had fun with it. I created a fun photo collage showing weekly pics I'd taken. The growth between weeks 12 and 15 was awfully impressive. Even though it was super short, I took great pleasure in attaching a bobby pin to the side of my head and declaring victory over it on social media. I could attach hair accessories again. Point awarded to … Fitz Koehler!

October 4. Friday.

I got zapped at an early morning radiation appointment, then jumped on a plane to Seattle, Washington, for our final DC Wonder Woman Run Series event of the year. I was eager to get back into my tutu and, since I had some hair, I was hoping I could wear my Wonder Woman tiara again. I had to trade it for a trucker cap back when I went bald for two reasons. First, because it hurt to wear it. Apparently, having lots of soft hair between a head and a crown is a good thing. And second, it looked really goofy on my cue ball noggin. Yes, I'm a grown-up who probably shouldn't get so excited about a tiara, but it was a special part of my Wonder Woman attire, and I really wanted to wear it again.

As usual, I reconnected with old buddies and also many new friends. I love it when people introduce themselves to me, especially if they mention that they listen to my podcast, use my Exact Formula for Weight Loss, or know me through running and social media. What could be more wonderful than meeting someone who shows up declaring they are already a fan of yours? It's very flattering. I feel honored to be integrated into so many exceptional lives. Even those of people I've never met. And when I do get to meet these new compadres, it thrills me to no end. Trust me when I say that I am as happy to meet you as you are to meet me. I've created lots of wonderful and long-lasting friendships with people I've met at running events, fitness presentations, and speaking engagements over the years. One of the most enviable aspects of my profession is my exposure to lovely people. Unfortunately, I'm often terrible with names, and chemo brain has made this issue far worse than usual. But if you can get past that, I ask that you please keep taking the time to greet me.

Speaking of quality humans, in Seattle, I had the great privilege of pouring some love on a sizey group of female first responders who ran our 5K in full uniform. We had firefighters, police officers, and military personnel on our course, and I gushed about them nonstop. I was also quick to take advantage of it being Breast Cancer Awareness Month. It was a bit spur of the moment, but I was able to whip up a compelling little presentation before I led everyone to the start line. On a whim, I invited all breast cancer patients and survivors to join me on our main stage. Once six or so joined, I gave a little history on myself and asked each woman to share her name, hometown, and how far out she was from treatment. Our audience cheered as each woman responded. I then encouraged everyone to get their annual exams and squeeze their stuff. Our crowd was supportive of the group and our messaging. And while I do this type of thing to inspire our athletes to change their behavior and do their exams, it's always encouraging and comforting to hear from women and men who've beaten the beast.

It's also worth mentioning that since I was in the Seattle area, I took the opportunity to sing the *Frasier* theme song at our finish line. Most folks had left by that time, but I sang the entire thing a la Kelsey Grammer and even threw in the "Good Night, Seattle" at the end. The remaining spectators seemed to have a good laugh at my nonsense, and fortunately, none of their ears were permanently damaged. If you were a fan of this 90s sitcom, then you know how cool that is.

I'm happy to share that I did wear my gold Wonder Woman tiara with the little red star in the front. Did it look fabulous? Probably not. But it didn't cause me any pain and, for the time being, that was good enough. Point awarded to … Fitz Koehler!

October 14. Monday.

I had spent the past week watching Ginger cheer at her high school homecoming events, getting zapped every day, and lying around with Stupid-Donkey-soaked washcloths on my chest. Preventing my skin from burning was a high priority, and I had done an excellent job so far. I was super itchy all of the time, but that seemed like a more tolerable alternative to blisters. On this day, I got to do both chemo #11 and radiation #32, which meant that the next day would be my very last radiation treatment. Yay!

October 15. Tuesday.

Since this was supposed to be a celebratory day with plenty of bell-ringing on the schedule, I decided to allow Ginger and Parker to miss school in the morning so that they could come along with Rob and me to my appointment. It was the first cancer related thing I had ever included them on, and I felt good about that. Before I woke up that morning, I hadn't thought that finishing up radiation would be such a big deal. For me, it wasn't a tumultuous process with miserable side effects like chemo had been, so I wasn't too anxious for it to be over. But when my alarm went off that morning, I was surprised that I actually did feel extra excited.

If you're unfamiliar, most cancer care facilities will honor the successful completion of each stage of treatment in some sort of jubilant way. For completion of radiation at TCC (The Cancer Center at North Florida), patients get to ring a big old bell with a long white rope that hangs from the clapper. The bell hangs on the wall of the large corridor patients trek through each day between the waiting room and the treatment area. Including my appointments with Dr. Hayes, I had walked past this big bell at least 80 times. While I could cruise by without giving it much thought on some days, on others, I just wanted to grab its clapper and bang it like Motley Crue's Tommy Lee on the drums. Trust me, I considered actually doing so many times. I mean, really. What would have happened? I wouldn't have been spanked or arrested. I probably wouldn't have been kicked out of radiation. I might have been given the stink eye though and an embarrassing scolding, so I was always able to repress those urges. But, today would be my day to bang that bell as aggressively as I wanted without getting in any sort of trouble. Perhaps good times did lay ahead!

As I checked in, all four Koehlers paused to enjoy some freshly baked radiation cookies. Yum! Morgan, Kayleigh, and Scott were in high spirits and we had some solid laughs while they were setting me up for the last time. Having such a delightful group of people to see throughout this process really was a godsend. The final painless zap took less than 15 minutes, and then it was time to celebrate. Before I left the room where the zapping took place, though, I invited Ginger in. In front of the massive zapper machine, we shot a fun little video dancing in unison to the song "The Git Up" by Blanco Brown, which we recorded on my phone using the TikTok app. Morgan did the filming. I was still wearing my blue hospital gown over my pink shorts, and I'm comfy telling you that this 15-second video was absolutely adorable. While our dancing was decent, all I see is joy whenever I watch it. Just a mother and daughter doing a victory dance over breast cancer. I shared the video via Facebook, Instagram, and Linkedin. It was received very enthusiastically across all channels, but it particularly caught fire on Linkedin where it was shared and viewed hundreds of thousands of times. People who work in oncology especially seemed to love it. Joyful celebrations are something the entire cancer community seems eager to bask in.

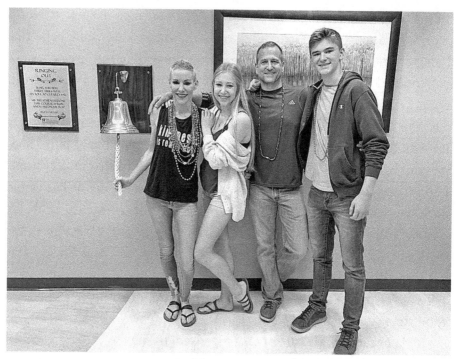

My bell ringing victory celebration with Ginger, Rob and Parker.
No more zaps!

Once we were done dancing, I changed back into my normal clothes and went to the big glorious bell, focused on hurting it. TCC treats all of their patients like they're the most important people in the world, and they specifically targeted me for a few extras. While I never waved my resume in anyone's face, word had gotten around about what I do professionally. Since my diagnosis, I had been invited to speak at a couple of their events. And that day they asked if their marketing team could record my bell ringing and do a little interview. I was happy to oblige.

I had already dropped 10 or so pounds, and was really on the thin side. I could see it in my face, which I didn't love, and I also had a weird black and blue spot on my cheek. This was likely due to my low platelet counts, which made me bruise easily. I had no idea how I ended up with one on my face, but mysterious circumstances were par for the course. I knew that whatever the high-definition cameras caught of me that day wasn't going to be gorgeous, but I chose not to let that bother me. I decided that I was a really good person going through a really hard experience, and that the best thing I could offer was a big smile on my oddly small and bruised face. In fact, with the volume of on-camera work I do, it would be outrageous to expect that I'd always look fabulous. People post terrible photos of me all the time, some with my mouth in a weird shape because I'm in the middle of talking and others with my eyes half-open. Looking a little off at a cancer care facility is probably more normal than not, so getting over myself was the right thing to do.

When I got to the bell, my sweet family, a plethora of administrators and nurses, and my radiation techs gathered around me. Dr. Hayes was out of town on business, but I'm sure she would have joined us too. Morgan led my little ceremony by reading a poem called "Ringing Out," which was written by Irve Le Moyne and appeared on the plaque next to the bell. She read it as it appeared:

RING THIS BELL
THREE TIMES WELL
ITS TOLL TO CLEARLY SAY

MY TREATMENT'S DONE
THIS COURSE IS RUN
AND I AM ON MY WAY

By this time, I was super excited, and I threw my left hand up in the air while ringing the hell out of that big bell with my right hand. I rang it far more than three times. I rang it in a way that would normally result in a bunch of cowboys and cattle showing up looking for a meal, hooting and hollering on the way. Everyone clapped and hugged, and after a brief video interview, we all walked away feeling like I had accomplished something fantastic. Apparently, I did. Point awarded to ... Fitz Koehler!

I was especially grateful to have my family by my side for this. They'd seen me so sick for so long, suffering so many harsh side effects. It was pretty fabulous for us to get together for a cancer-related event that was victorious. Another point awarded to .... the Koehler family!

October 19. Saturday.

Dr. Hayes asked me to host a Zumbathon fundraiser, the profits of which would go to the local Making Strides Against Breast Cancer event. The Zumbathon took place in the giant lobby of the cancer center and was organized by Whitney Perkins, another radiology oncologists' wife. She's a spunky little thing and did a superior job getting 10 different Zumba instructors signed up to alternate teaching funky dance work-outs to 45-plus participants. Our guests donated funds in exchange for the opportunity to participate. While I still wasn't down with wearing pink ribbons, I've never been unmotivated to support the American Cancer Society or contribute. I was more than thrilled to give back to a cause that worked tirelessly to take care of cancer patients like me. My work was uncomplicated, which made for a relaxed afternoon. I started the event by welcoming all participants and sharing a bit about my breast cancer experience. Then I gave some guidelines for the day and proceed-ed to introduce each energetic Zumba instructor as he or she took the stage. As you can imagine, these instructors were lively and saucy and I enjoyed watching everyone, including my sweet Ginger Bean, shake their booties and boobies and anything else they could get to wiggle with them. I praised each instructor on whatever they did best after their two to three songs' worth of instruction. Then I'd get folks pumped up for the next instructor. One of the best things about being on the micro-phone is my power to publicly pour love on people. It's one thing to think that someone is wonderful and share that in private. It's quite another to be able to proclaim someone's awesomeness via a professional sound system. Helping people feel special and proud is one of the things I'm compelled to do, and I revel in watching them respond to kind remarks.

The only odd thing about the day was my inability to participate. I was still fairly tired and weak from chemo, my tummy was irritable, and my left boob was far too sore for bouncing. In fact, that's something I was surprised by. The effect radiation had on my breast tissue, paired with the remaining sensitivity from surgery, made for one sore boob. My skin only looked slightly pink, but if we could have peered inside me, I imagined that all of my soft tissue would look black and blue. It felt as though my left breast and rib cage had been beaten with a bat. As I sat on the sidelines, I thought back to the days when I was teaching fitness classes and about how often I used to be the fittest person in the room. Sure, it was strange to not feel that way, but it was all for a good reason, and I was 100% confident I would come back stronger when my treatments were done.

October 26. Saturday.

After a stress-free week without any treatment appointments, my family and I attended the Making Strides Against Breast Cancer fundraising 5K. Put on by the local branch of the American Cancer Society (ACS), all money would go toward the Hope Lodge of Gainesville, which provides a free place for cancer patients and their families to stay while undergoing medical treatment. It's a great cause, and I experienced firsthand the benefit of living close to all of my medical care; I definitely wanted to support others who needed the same. The executive director of the ACS had reached out several weeks earlier to see if I would be the keynote speaker for the event. I was more than happy to do so. Since I spent the majority of my time announcing races, supporting amazing people, and pushing causes in *other towns*, I thought it would be awesome to invite my local people to do something great in *my* hometown. And it was. Through online donations, I was able to raise about $2,000 and also put together a wonderful group of friends to come out and walk with Team Fitzness. I think we had about 30 on my team, and I was proud of that: friends, neighbors, family members, online friends and Ginger's high school cheerleading team. Oh! And Piper also came out, sporting pink necklaces that made our team look extra cute.

While I didn't don any pink ribbons, I did wear my custom hot pink Fitzness tank top and a royal blue running skirt with big white stars on it. Before the walk began, everyone gathered in the courtyard of the posh local outdoor shopping center. My friend, and local radio personality, Storm Roberts was the emcee. He introduced me with high praise, and

I very much appreciated it. Storm is superb at what he does, and he's a cancer survivor as well.

While I never want cancer to define me, I do enjoy talking about it. What I don't enjoy talking about *yet* is my personal experience with cancer. Mind you, I do it really well, and I know it. I just don't enjoy it yet. When I start talking about me and referencing my hardships, I feel weird things happen in my chest area. Not my boobs. My heart. It beats a little faster and my breath tries to escape me. I also become squirmy inside my own skin. My cool, calm demeanor starts to dissipate and I have to fight to regain it. I've spent my entire career talking about others and ways they can live better and longer. It's been fairly difficult to talk about myself and about having to face cancer. For a girl who speaks for a living, it's an unusual conundrum. In fact, while I can talk about running or fitness without ever spitting out an "um" or an "ahh," I almost instantly stammer a bit when the topic turns to me. I turn it around within the first 60 seconds, but it's something I'm going to have to work on.

Once I took the stage, it took me about 30 seconds to gather myself before I started to hit it out of the park. I was able to tell a miniature version of my tale and motivate the audience to squeeze their stuff. I also asked them to recognize and celebrate the many breast cancer survivors and patients in our midst and publicly gave thanks to my family and my extraordinary medical teams from FCS and TCC. TCC brought out a sizable squad, including Dr. Hayes, and it was meaningful to be able to show my appreciation for them in front of our very large audience. My presentation lasted about 10 minutes and, when I was done, I walked off the stage to fantastic applause. When I returned the microphone to Storm, he suggested that someone make a T-shirt with "Squeeze Your Stuff" on it. Within a few minutes, a woman ran up to me, telling me she was going to make those T-shirts. I'm still waiting for mine. I was excited by the opportunity to do this more often. I was able to add light and levity to a tough subject while still imploring people to take action toward their own health. I was committed to continuing to make noise on behalf of cancer causes moving forward.

Once we hit the start line, we paused for a team photo and then took off for our 5K walk. Remember, this wasn't a race at all. Running wasn't even encouraged. This was simply a big walk for fundraising and awareness and, because of that, people who might have been intimidated by a running race felt comfortable taking part. As we started moving I felt great, still riding high from the adrenaline my presentation provided. However, that all disappeared within a half-mile. My body revolted and I feared I might have to puke and then quit walking altogether. That was going to be a bummer. I kept walking and thinking about what a disappointment it would be if the spunky little speaker in the skirt had to tap out. I don't know why nausea hit me the way it did, but I suppose that's just how Godzilla was going to play it that day. Fortunately, I was able to drink water, slow down, and keep going. Walking with my neighbor, Laurie, who was an oncology nurse, seemed to be my crutch in case I went down quickly. I didn't. I was able to walk the entire course and went home feeling proud and productive.

Fitzness Log

My workouts were delightfully consistent and I was making progress with my weightlifting. That's one of the things I love about strength training — you can easily track your progress. Can you lift more weight or do more reps? If the answer is yes, you're doing the right thing! I had been dying to swim but was advised against it during radiation. Apparently swimming can dry your skin, which could lead to more irritation. Once I had rung that bell though, I was able to dive right in. Except, I didn't dive. I casually walked into the little warm pool at my gym.

I started getting in the warm pool for a good 60 minutes almost daily. I'd bring my favorite aqua strength training tools and just move my body in a variety of ways. The warm pool crowd was composed of senior citizens who loved to chat and tell stories, so I made a bunch of interesting new friends while I exercised. My new squad showed up every day purely to enhance their quality of life. They knew that if they wanted to keep pains at bay and continue with vibrancy, they needed to exercise. I wish more young adults had the same respect for health.

Chapter 11

Mascots and Mosh Pits

November 1. Friday.

Chemo #12 was absolutely uneventful, which was a good thing. At this point, many side effects of the mean chemo were waning. There were no more crazy rashes on my face or chest. The bottom half of my finger and toenails looked healthier, and that rotten stench was gone (thank goodness). The painful green alien sludge had disappeared from under my scalp and my quads no longer felt like I was climbing Mt. Everest every day. While the hair on my head was growing fairly slowly, I had it and that was worth celebrating. I also had leg and arm hair, which I wasn't dancing about, but also didn't mind. Sadly, I only had an itsy bitsy showing of nostril hair, and my nose still ran like a leaky faucet. I still think it's peculiar, yet hilarious that I've spent a chunk of my life wishing for nostril hair. What the hell?

November 6. Wednesday.

Feeling fairly decent, I was stoked to board my plane for Monterey, California. I'm bonkers over the place, people, and being part of this race weekend. It's put on by the Big Sur Marathon Foundation, which also organizes the Big Sur International Marathon (BSIM) each April. Rudy and I have the privilege of announcing their two largest events each year, and I can comfortably confess that I pinch myself because of it. They are that good. Since any sort of leisurely activity had been off of my agenda for a long time, I decided to fly in a day early for some pre-race rest and relaxation.

November 7. Thursday.

When Rudy arrived we had some fun in a spunky Jeep Wrangler that he rented. As an aside, before I had Ginger, I drove a Wrangler, and it brought me infinite joy. Presently, I drive a Jeep Cherokee. It's a fine car, indeed. But since my quality of life has been diminished so much during my year of breast cancer treatment, I'm looking to compensate for the losses in a big way. My intention is to purchase another Wrangler when I'm done.

Friends, quality of life matters a lot. Living is not just about how much time we get on earth, it's about doing things that fill us up with joy and finding the fabulous in each moment. And it's also about being with people who bring us happiness. When asked what I want for special events like Christmas and my birthday, tangible items rarely make my list. I traditionally choose to ask for adventures instead. I would much rather partake in water sports, zip-line, or attend a cool concert than receive something in a box. However, I can confidently say that driving a Jeep Wrangler with the roof off turns up my happiness volume to level 10. It makes every moment driving from point A to point B a cheery and adventurous one. My next Wrangler will be brightly-colored and have a manual transmission since driving stick shift is extra fun. So when chemo is done, and Dr. Gordan sends me off into the world again, you will find me on the backroads in a filthy, but fabulous Wrangler.

Back to Monterey. While running the Big Sur International Marathon course is a big deal, driving the course is also a fabulous thing to do. Rudy and I build that into our schedule every time we announce the Monterey Bay Half Marathon (MBHM). Running across the Bixby Bridge is one of the highlights of the BSIM, and by golly, I decided to make it a highlight of our day trip. Sort of. I'll preface this by telling you that even though running the BSIM sounds like a magical experience, I hope I never get to do it. Why? Because that would mean that I wouldn't be announcing the race, which brings me far more joy than running ever could. If you haven't done the math yet, there are only a few things on the planet I'd choose to do over announcing my races. And those few things revolve around Ginger and Parker.

We pulled in on the north side of the Bixby Bridge where there's a spot for tourists to park and take photos. The plan was to get out and enjoy the scenic views, but traffic was light and I was feeling cheeky. I jumped on the opportunity to run about 25% of the way across the bridge and back while Rudy took pictures. I kept my steps as light as possible, trying not to bounce "leftie" too much, and I threw my hands up in the air as though I was winning some sort of race. Obviously. That's how winners roll. The pictures ended up being really cute and now I can claim (with proof) that I have run on Bixby Bridge.

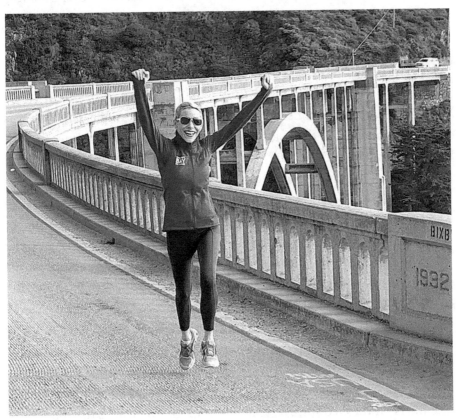

Running across the Bixby Bridge. Just because I could. Go me!

The other fun thing we did on our drive was stop to loiter. Yes, you read that right. We stopped to loiter, and it wasn't the first time. See, there's this very arbitrary sign out in the middle of nowhere in front of fenced-in private property, of which there is no structure, that states, "No Loitering." Now, when I see one of those signs in front of a gas station in a busy city, I don't give it a second thought. Loiterers could definitely be a problem in a place like that. But whenever I see this particular sign in this particular place, I wonder. What the hell prompted this? Who drove 20 miles away from society, parked in a desolate place, and just hung out in front of this dude's fence? I can't fathom. So, whenever we go, we pull over in a weird place, get out, and go photograph ourselves loitering in front of that sign. We pose with our arms crossed leaning up against the fence looking bored, sitting, and pondering. Sometimes we go as far as to lie down in the dirt. The photos were absolutely hilarious. After finishing our drive, we paused in Carmel-By-the-Sea to peruse expensive stores we had no business shopping in. It was fun to be out doing leisurely things, and I enjoyed every minute of it.

November 8. Friday.

While we always consider this event weekend unique, this one was extra special because the prior year, we had to cancel our half marathon. Smoke from the horrific 2018 "Camp" fire had turned our direction and was doomed to leave a dangerous layer of smog over our event. Having athletes run in those conditions would be akin to having them stop to smoke an entire cigarette every half mile. That was a health risk no respectable race organization could support. The decision was made the evening before the race by Doug Thurston, under the guidance of his medical director and the local weather expert. I was tasked with sharing the sad news of our cancellation at the expo, which was still packed with runners, vendors, and volunteers. Surprisingly, it was an emotionally challenging thing to do. The pragmatic side of me had been thinking, "People are burning alive in their cars up the road; canceling a race is not such a big deal!" But when I got on the microphone, turned down the music and asked for everyone's attention, my heart sank. Suddenly, disappointing all of these wonderful people who had paid for, trained for, traveled to, and poured their hearts into our race, had become quite upsetting. I made the announcement in a way that allowed people to walk away feeling good about the decision to cancel, but many people were sad and rightfully disappointed. This year, most of those athletes had returned, and the excitement was palpable.

Rudy and I basked in the lovefest that took place when we reunited with our BSMF family. They were particularly concerned about me back in April during the marathon weekend, so it felt good to show up with a little bit of hair and a big smile on my face. We took turns announcing the expo and then headed to the VIP party that evening for sponsors and special guests. I was a little tired, so I hung back a bit during the party and left early. I knew I needed to get to bed to be at my best for our races.

November 9. Saturday.

Rudy and I started our day with the Pacific Grove Lighthouse 5K and By-the-Bay 3K. These events launch in a beautiful park called *Lover's Point* and are perfect for entire family units to participate in. I was feeling mostly good with decent energy and was looking forward to an action-packed day. But the cold was a real bear that morning. Temperatures were in the low 40s, and the wind was fierce. We were steps away from the ocean, and if I had long hair again it would have been blowing all over my face. While I always show up to my events thinking that I'm dressed appropriately, I rarely get it right. I was wearing leggings, a T-shirt, a cropped sweatshirt, and gloves. Sounds good, right? Nope. Not good at all. The real problem here was that I had to balance dressing properly for cold weather while also dressing attractively. I work on stages for crying out loud! I can't show up looking dumpy or frumpy. So there lies my predicament, and I almost always get it wrong. This leads me to find other ways to stay warm. Sometimes I coerce people into hugging, cuddling, or holding my hands, and sometimes I get even more creative. Per usual, we arrived way too early and our suffering from the elements was real, so I decided to take action and hide underneath the table on our stage. It was covered with a big heavy tablecloth that blocked the wind nicely. I found it to be a fabulous little shelter for a good 20 minutes or so. Runners were only trickling in at that point, so no one was exposed to my nonsense, which to me felt a tad genius. I've hidden under tables before, and I'll do it again.

Once the national anthem ended, Rudy stayed at the main stage, and I led the athletes over to the start line to get our races underway. There were a handful of serious runners up at the front of our start line with one young man trying to break a world record for his age group, but the rest of our pack seemed delightfully unserious and highly motivated to have fun. Since they exclusively run on a road that parallels the ocean, I always encourage them to keep an eye on the sea for whale breaches and whale tails. During November, this area is packed with humpback whales, blue whales, gray whales, fin whales, orca (killer whales) and dolphins. In previous races, we've often found ourselves at the finish line, wondering where the heck all of our runners were. Turns out, they stopped to watch a bunch of whales launching themselves over the water. Cool, right? And because of that, I often ask Doug if he will summon the whales on the microphone before I yell "GO." Being a good sport and having grown accustomed to my antics, Doug now obliges my request with animated whale noises. Think "Dory" in the movie *Finding Nemo*. It's classic.

Since we had thousands of participants, we broke them up into corrals at the start. I yelled "GO" about a dozen times, and each corral ended up being more silly and rowdy than the last. They had no idea that they were filling my heart up with sparkly rainbow-colored happy juice. Do you know what I'm saying? For all of the horrible hardships I'd had to endure through my cancer treatments, standing at the helm of such spirited crowds was the ultimate way to refill my tank and make me feel whole again. When I asked something preposterous like, "Is anyone trying to qualify for the Olympic games today?" and thousands of people shouted in response, it was healing. Runners have been my best medicine.

Our finish line was just as entertaining as the start with the majority of our participants throwing their hands up high or celebrating in their own unique way. At the start line I had given them all strict orders to honor their finishes with some spunk, and they did. Once we wrapped things up at Lover's Point, Rudy and I went back to the expo so I could teach my Strength Training for Runners clinic.

I have to commend the BSMF for their efforts on their speaker series, because not all race organizations do it well. Doug starts by choosing high-quality speakers, which goes a long way. And then his team does a fine job of marketing our presentations. Sometimes races will bring in speakers and do little to nothing to notify participants. That's just a waste of resources. BSMF does not mess around, and because of that, my rooms are always packed. I live for standing-room-only style crowds, and that's exactly what I get when I'm in Monterey. Hordes of motivated people show up to learn, and I love it.

I always arrive early to make small talk and get to know my audience before my presentation actually starts. I do this on the microphone so everyone can hear, and it's a wise way to get people engaged, relaxed, and eager to participate. I find out where they are from, which races they're participating in, and much more. And we laugh. We laugh before, during, and after my presentations. My mission is to make fitness understandable, attainable, and fun. When people show up to hear me speak, I know they are going to be far more engaged if I am actually entertaining. If they are hanging on every word I say, anticipating the next laugh, they're probably going to be absorbing far more of the science and smarty-pants stuff I'm dishing out. This specific audience was particularly responsive.

Once I got started, I did a light-hearted 60-second breast cancer/squeeze your stuff deal, warned them that because of chemo-brain I may need help with a few words, and moved on. Fortunately, I was able to pull up all of my words and didn't require any lifelines. Something funny did happen in the middle of my talk, though. I had just finished discussing proprioception and balance training. Proprioception, also known as the "6th sense," is your body's instinctive ability to adjust and stay upright when your balance is tested. The more time you put into balance training, the better your proprioception will be and the less likely you are to fall down. Make sense? Good. I had just finished teaching that little lesson while standing on the front edge of my stage, which was about a couple of feet off the ground. I don't know how it happened, but I took a step to the left, and ended up unintentionally stepping off of it. As this happened, I waved my arms around like cartoon characters do when they're about to fall off a building. The audience gasped loudly, and all I could think about was how awful it was going to be when the noisy lady going through chemo wiped out in front of everyone. Could I *be* any more pathetic? Luckily, I didn't wipe out. I hit the ground in an unsteady way, but I was able to stick the landing enough to remain upright. In a little stroke of genius, I immediately threw my arms up in the air like a gymnast and shouted "proprioception!" The crowd roared laughing.

When my one-hour time slot was over, I wrapped things up and offered to stay outside the room to meet people and answer more questions if anyone had them. It's possible that 100% of my audience took me up on my offer. Some folks actually had follow-up questions, but many just wanted to share a hug or take a photo together. Getting to personally meet so many of our participants tends to pay off on race day and beyond. I'm often able to pull up these individuals from memory and give them a personalized shout out at our start and finish lines. And I frequently form long-term friendships this way. It's a win-win for us both.

November 10. Sunday.

Redemption time. The vast majority of our athletes were those who'd been turned away the year prior. Yes, we sold out and had lots of extra athletes with us, but to suggest that people were cranked up to run this race would be a dramatic understatement. Rudy and I jumped on our microphones at least an hour before start time and enjoyed every minute of our pre-race pandemonium. Heck! We were also really pumped up about this year. Like everyone else last year, we were robbed of announcing one of our favorite events. It hurt our hearts big time. Team Noisy welcomed about 9,000 athletes into the Noisy Nation that morning because they were not being quiet! We like our start lines rowdy, but everyone brought a little extra crazy to the Monterey Bay Half Marathon in 2019.

Our finish line was equally raucous, as even the elite runners celebrated their finishes in a lively way. In many races, the speedsters often seem a little bored or nonplussed, even when they win an event. That did not happen in Monterey. And other than a bit of pain in my low back, I was having an incredible morning. Rudy and I danced our booties off for hours and the crowds boogied too. Throughout our hectic day, the BSMF team continued to pour love and concern on me. Blue Jacket Claudia Campbell, who never comes to the finish line, came over to check on me and bring refreshments. She'd been

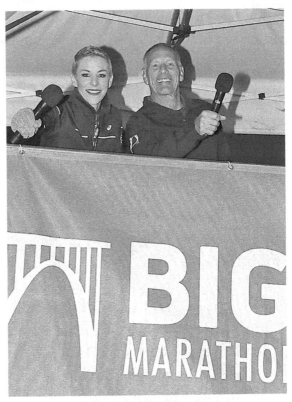

In the tall tower with Rudy.
Photo by BSMF

mothering me all weekend, and I loved it. Blue Jackets Megan O'Neill and Joe Vargo also brought us some treats. In fact, I could provide a long list of team member names who stopped what they were doing that morning to come to our stage and make sure I was okay. For them to do that during such a busy event truly made me feel loved.

The lovefest continued at our annual post-race High Five Dinner, which was held back at Ferrante's, exclusively for staff and Blue Jackets. I'd say we had about 75 attendees. In celebration of a successful weekend, we passed a microphone around to anyone who wanted to share a fond memory, humorous story, or praise from the weekend. I looked forward to hearing everyone's short presentations as most are either really sweet or really comical. In particular, I'm always eager to hear from Doug who has a bone dry sense of humor and a terrific ability to tell tales. He normally goes first since he hosts the dinner, so I can't tell you how surprised I was by how he started things out. I was sad that he skipped his traditionally hilarious stories, but flabbergasted when he opted to tell everyone that the best thing about his weekend was, "Seeing Fitz Koehler show up happy and looking healthy." I'm pretty sure everyone else stood up and clapped in response, but all of the water in my eyes made it difficult to see clearly. Throughout all of the stressful, scary, and painful moments I've endured because of breast cancer, this exemplified how there was always another quality human trying to make up the difference. Was getting on planes and zig-zagging the country a tough thing to do while undergoing treatment? Absolutely. Was it in my best interest? You bet your life it was.

When it was my turn on the microphone, I took the opportunity to do two things. First, I had to lay high praise on the other half of Team Noisy. Rudy deserved credit for his big voice, happy attitude, and robust ability to get things done. He also deserved kudos for debuting his twerking skills at the half marathon, which almost made me roll off our stage laughing. I think it all started because he was bending down awkwardly to pick something up. When I saw his butt leaning out toward me, I publicly declared, "OMG! Rudy is twerking!" And instead of waving me off, he went with it, and dove into his version of the twerk. I wish I had caught it on video because it was spectacular. Rudy's booty was jutting out in all directions while his arms were doing something else completely. As you can imagine, everyone loved hearing about his funky moves. The second thing I did was share my humble appreciation for the endless amounts of concern, love, and efforts by my friends in the room. I acknowledged the "I'm so happy you're alive" hugs that said, "I need to give you a good squeeze to make sure you're really still here." Truth be told, I started off the year downright fearful for my life. Those long, hard hugs meant just as much to me and I was infinitely grateful to be with so many dear friends. Once I let them know how much they meant to me, I passed on the microphone.

November 11. Monday.

Ouch. Remember how I mentioned that I ended up with some severe low back issues because of all of my muscle loss? This was the first time that happened. My L5 disk was freaking out and I was left roaming through airports slightly bent over and having the wind knocked out of me with every step. It was excruciating. However, I discovered something new on the trip home. I rarely drank alcohol before I was diagnosed, but had sworn it off completely once I started being pumped with bags of poison. Combining the two couldn't be wise, now could it? In extreme pain at the airport, I decided to give it a go. Maybe a couple of beers would help? Maybe liquor? Well, throughout my long day in the air, I consumed two beers and two gin and tonics. Sadly, none of it dulled my pain. But none of it made me sick either. Apparently I was open for business and going to allow myself the occasional beer or cocktail if I wanted. Cheers to that!

Back home the next day, I crawled around the floor in agony and eventually got Dr. Gordan to call in a prescription for steroids. They, combined with physical therapy, got me back upright within a few days. Good thing, because I was announcing another large event the following weekend. When I started with chemo, I definitely expected stomach problems and hair loss. I had absolutely no clue that every time I stood up, there would be another seemingly obscure side effect trying to knock me down. I literally felt like one of those Bozo the Clown Bop Bags. I'd get whacked. I'd go down and BAM! I'd spring back up. The back and forth was mentally exhausting, but the effort was always worth it. The carrots dangling in front of me — my kids and my races— always inspired me to bounce back. Come hell or high water, I wasn't going to miss out on either.

November 15. Friday.

Feeling significantly better, I enthusiastically loaded up my car with a portable electric stimulation device attached to my back. It was keeping my muscles mostly calm and I would wear it all weekend as I worked. I was driving two hours south of my home to announce the St. Pete

Run Fest weekend with Rob, Parker, and his best friend, Kayla. This was my only race announcing job in Florida for the entire year and it was a doozy. The owners/race directors are brothers, Keith and Ryan Jordan. They put on a high-quality event weekend full of fun extras and tons of support from sponsors. Our start line, finish line, and festival areas are right next to a gorgeous harbor full of boats. The whole thing is very Florida. Except for the weather that weekend. It was obnoxiously and oddly cold.

Making up for the rude temperatures, though, was the fact that my good friend and fellow Florida Gator, John Pelkey, was going to be announcing with me. I recommended John to fill in for me when I had a scheduling conflict, and they quickly fell in love with him. In a stroke of luck, we were both free that year, so they hired us to work together. John and I had been looking forward to it since we confirmed the dates, but the reality of our pairing was even better than expected. Our very bold and sarcastic personalities meshed perfectly on our microphones and we laughed our fool heads off the entire weekend. Thankfully, our audiences did too. We had athletes and spectators buckled over laughing nonstop,

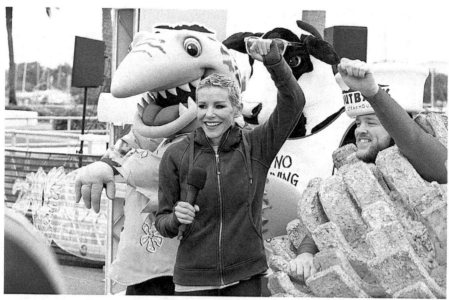

Mascot dance party! Photo by BBActionPhoto.com

and that included Ryan Jordan. While we love a nice paycheck, it's pretty rewarding when your boss keeps coming over to tell you how much he's enjoying your efforts.

Each race within the St. Pete Run Fest had its own element of fabulosity, but I'd like to tell you about some of my personal highlights. I'll start with our surprise request during the start of the Outback Steakhouse 5K Saturday morning. While John and I were instructing and entertaining our athletes at the start line, a man in a giant Bloomin' Onion costume approached to tell us that he was ready to lead the Outback cheer. Ummm. This was not in our script. Where did this guy come from? Turning the microphone over to a big Bloomin' Onion seemed like a pretty bad idea. What kind of expertise or talent could a giant crispy appetizer have to bestow? The costumed man did have a cute face, but we had no reason to trust his performance skills. However, since Outback Steakhouse had probably forked over a ton of cash to be the title sponsor, John and I relented. I remember bringing that big tasty dish up onto our stage and gathering everyone's attention, expecting whatever was going to happen next to be an awkward fail. Instead, it was pure delight. Mr. Onion used his big voice to lead everyone in a chant and, shockingly, everyone went along with it.

Aussie, Aussie, Aussie. Oy! Oy! Oy!

Aussie, Aussie, Aussie. Oy! Oy! Oy!

Aussie, Aussie, Aussie. Oy! Oy! Oy!

We had thousands of people chanting along enthusiastically, and I was instantly smitten with Mr. Onion. His confidence and spunk were pretty cool to witness, and this would not be our last rendezvous. The next time I saw Mr. Onion would be at our official Mascot Race.

This is a list of the exceptionally intimidating group of athletes that were competing in the Mascot Race and who they were representing:

- Cow - Chick-fil-A
- Pete the Pelican -Tampa Bay Rowdies
- Rocky the Bull - The University of South Florida
- Raymond Ray - Tampa Bay Rays

- Salty the Pelican - The St. Pete Run Fest
- Bloomin' Onion - Outback Steakhouse
- Phinley the Thresher Shark - Clearwater Threshers

We held this exciting mascot race right before the start of our kids' races. The crowds were huge, and since the mascots made their way to the start line quite a bit early, we had no choice but to kick things off by finding out who had the best dance moves. There was lots of feathered-flapping from our pelicans, thrusting by the Thresher Shark, muscle moves from Rocky, and a surprising amount of twerking by Mr. Onion. Who knew? Obviously, the cow had great mooves as well. (I know. I know. Puns are so bad.) I hate to brag, but this is where I shine. When races are faced with delays or significant gaps of space to fill, I pounce on opportunities to engage with the crowds or promote silliness. The mascot dance party was not in our script or on the schedule. However, we had tons of people lining our course waiting to be entertained. So I just boldly declared, "It's time for the mascot dance party!" That's one of the most rewarding and empowering benefits that come along with being in control of the microphone: when I tell people to do something, they usually do it. None of our mascots checked with their handlers for a schedule or contract change. They simply broke it down and got funky. And, oh, they could dance! They fed into all of the popular dance moves the kids were obsessed with at the time. They were dabbing, flossing, moonwalking, doing the Douggie, the Whoa, and more. And I danced with them. After a grueling year, I was elated to be out in the middle of the course, giggling nonstop as the crowds of children and parents cheered.

Back to the mascot race. It was heated. Lots of elbows and tail fins and feathers were flying, but Pelican Pete flew through the finish line first. After taking several breaks on our 100-yard course, the Chick-fil-A cow pulled up the rear. For the record, I had been looking forward to our mascot race since I was booked for this event. I wish more of my race organizations did this. (Hint, hint, to my other race directors.) This is quality entertainment!

Highlight #2 also came from a costumed individual, but this time that person was warming up and wearing a race bib at the front of our half marathon start line. Usually, we reserve the space closest to the actual start line for our very fastest runners. The slower a runner or walker's pace, the further back they line up to start the race. Again, this is done to create a comfortable flow and so faster people don't slam into the backs of the slower people or get stuck struggling to weave around them. John and I looked at each other and silently agreed that this person in a head-to-toe furry lion costume should not have been up at the front. We had no clue exactly who was inside that bulky getup, but we didn't think that the lion should have been where he or she was. We couldn't wait to see that lion limp in with its head off toward the end of the day. Once the lion came in, we'd learn the name, gender, and hometown of that person.

Fast forward to the finish line. John and I had just welcomed our half marathon champion, who finished at 1:11:57. We were continuing to make a stink over the next few speedsters when "Oh! Nooooo! We can't believe it! It's the lion! No waaaaay!" As we simultaneously looked down at our announcer laptop to discover the lion's name, all we saw was - First Name: Master, Last Name: Lion! Master Lion got his name called in enthusiastic unison by his two mesmerized announcers, and the crowds went wild. John and I were in disbelief. He finished at 1:24:48, 10th overall. And yes, we were able to see that he did cross all of the timing mats during his 13.1-mile dash. He did not cut the course or cheat. The 35-year-old Australian dude inside that furry costume was just one hell of an athlete, and one hell of a silly guy. In fact, post-race, we discovered each other on Instagram, he's @masterlionofficial, and it turns out that Master Lion runs races in his full fuzzy getup quite often. He posted a pic with John and me on November 18, 2019. Go check him out.

Highlight #3. I can't tell you how happy it makes me when my family runs the races I announce. Because my events are scattered across America, it only happens a handful of times each year. But it's gratifying for all of us when things line up. Rob, Parker, and Kayla signed up for the 5K, as well as our chosen family members, Susan Regalado and her adult son, Joey. For the record, Ginger didn't join us because she was occupied with cheerleading camp. Susan is in her sixties, has had FIVE hip replacement surgeries, and had "walking a 5K that Fitz announces" on her bucket list. She's always been very spunky, and she recruited her doting son, Joey, 29, to participate with her.

At the start of the Outback Steakhouse 5K, they all lined up together in the back of the pack, which was appropriate for their pace. Sometimes I think my kids do that to avoid being recognized by mom. Yeah right. As if I'd let Parker off the hook because I couldn't see him behind the other 5,000 athletes. I took the opportunity to acknowledge all five of them, and share a bit about Susan and her efforts to overcome five hip replacement surgeries, which made everyone cheer. And then I told them that my handsome 14-year-old son, Parker, was lined up in the back, and it was my duty to embarrass him. "So if everyone wouldn't mind turning toward the back of the pack and shouting 'Hi Parker,' I'd really appre-

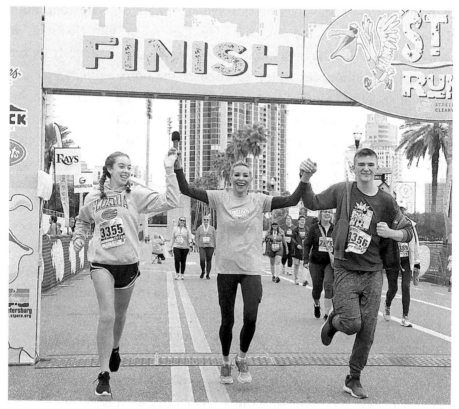

Running Kayla and Parker through the finish. Photo by BBActionPhoto.com

ciate it." On the count of three, they gave out the biggest "Hiiiii Parker" that ever lived. You could hear it a hundred miles away, and I beamed with pride. Fortunately, my kids seem to actually enjoy that embarrassing mom stuff. It's part of the deal when they run a race and mom is on the microphone.

Kayla and Parker leisurely walked the 5K, but still finished somewhere in between first and last place. Rob, Joey, and Susan, on the other hand, were dead last and received the warmest welcome of the day. Apparently, she kept joking about cutting the course during their journey, and the boys had to keep nudging her along. I was immensely proud of her and cherished the opportunity to personally escort her across the finish line. It's always enjoyable when I do that for strangers, but sharing this kind of moment with family is incomprehensibly special. On the flip side, Rob ran the half marathon the next day and just scooted on by me with not much more than a little wave. I guess he was on a mission.

Before I finish telling you about the St. Pete Run Fest, I must pause to rave about John Pelkey. I'm a bit of a snob when it comes to working with other announcers as I've been pampered by the chemistry I share with Rudy. As a rule, I only want to be part of teams that can deliver extraordinary energy and professionalism to our events. Trust me. I've worked with wonderful humans whom I really liked personally who were just very flat on the microphone, and the outcomes have been painful. People who drone on reading scripts and stats as though they are a TV commentator instead of in front of a live audience are killjoys. Working with people who do that makes me look bad too. I've tried to compensate for low-energy partners, but it's almost impossible to make up for the difference. On the flip side, I knew that working with John would be electric, and I couldn't wait to collaborate with him. His big booming voice is magnificent, as are his comedic abilities. If he were to perform a stand-up routine at a comedy club, I'd be the first customer at the door. I've enjoyed being a runner at races he's announced in the past, and working side-by-side with him was even better. He was the best I'd ever heard him on the microphone, and he danced with me for hours. As a reminder, I spent the entire weekend wearing a portable electric stimulation device on my back. It could have been really rough. Instead, John kept me laughing nonstop. Fingers crossed that we will get to announce many more races together in the future. And also: Go Gators!

November 21. Thursday.

After a fairly busy week, which included a special MUGA scan to test how well my heart was beating, I was up at 4 a.m. to fly to The City of Brotherly Love. By this time, Rob was looking far less concerned as I ventured off toward TSA. The AACR Philadelphia Marathon weekend was exciting for a variety of reasons. It was a massive event with more than 30,000 athletes, and this was the first time I'd be announcing it. I was pursued that summer and hired by the title sponsor, The American Association for Cancer Research (AACR). They were hoping to bring more energy to the start and finish lines of the marathon, along with more attention to the AACR. Who better to do that than the highly energetic professional race announcer who just happened to be battling cancer at the moment? No one! I was looking forward to announcing this monster event while doing something positive for a cause that was near and dear to my heart. While I'm certainly happy to support the definite cure and, hopefully, a vaccine for breast cancer, it is very satisfying to pitch in and help find solutions for all types of cancers. My heart has been broken at the hand of pancreatic, skin, and blood cancers alone. The AACR is dedicated to accelerating the conquest of cancer. Partnering up to support the AACR, which is the first and largest cancer research organization in America, felt great.

When I arrived in chilly Philadelphia around 11 a.m., I was eager to get to my hotel, dump my stuff, and go sightseeing. My passion for my country has always been immense, and I was excited to hit the streets and saturate myself in some American history. I was bubbling with excitement as I walked up to see the Liberty Bell. I've traveled the world and have seen some extraordinary things, but I learned about the Liberty Bell when I was in first grade. Getting up close and personal with it genuinely made me giddy. Sure, it's just a bell. But, it symbolizes so much for those of us devoted to freedom. Plus, that big crack is big-time intriguing. A selfie with the Liberty Bell was the perfect start to my weekend. Then I took a tour of Independence Hall, where the US Declaration of Independence and Constitution were debated and adopted. I felt starstruck as I sat in the moderate-size building where the titans of freedom came together to craft documents that would form the greatest country in the world. Squeal! Do I sound like a nerd? Probably. Do I care? Not even a little. Some folks get dorky over actors, athletes, and musicians. I do so for the Founding Fathers. Swoon!

I also met up with my new friend and runner Marc Kassel, who I'd met in the Atlanta airport on our way to Philly. He was taking on the Freedom Challenge and running all three races that weekend. The half marathon, the 8K, and the marathon. While this may sound completely bonkers to many of you reading this, and it is, Marc was just one of over 1,000 athletes who registered to do the challenge. These challenges are a popular thing in the running world, and this guy doesn't know how to say "no" to them. Marc and I visited Ben Franklin's grave and then toured the Constitution Museum together. Having a buddy to do a little sightseeing with turned out to be a really pleasant surprise. I'm no stranger to traveling and touring alone, but this new friendship was a cool addition to my adventure.

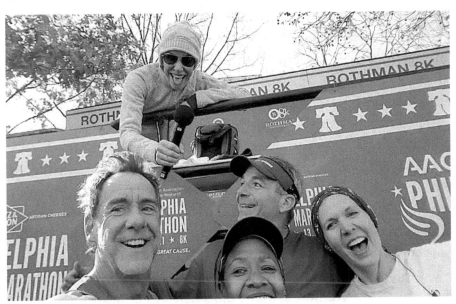

Fun with some Boston Buddies. Photo by Marty Clark

That evening I went to the official VIP party, which was held to acknowledge special guests and sponsors. Our van of running industry notables included Meb Keflezighi, an American Olympian who took silver in the marathon in Athens, 2004. He won the New York City Marathon in 2009 and earned his official spot in American hearts in 2014 when he won the Boston Marathon, the year after the horrific bombing. Yes. Meb has a long accomplished history as a world-class distance runner. However, I'm pretty sure most people adore him because of his charisma and kindness. Meb and I had both been at the Los Angeles Marathon together several times, but never really crossed paths. It was a pleasure to get to know him on a personal level. He's an easy-going guy who seems not to accept his position on a pedestal. Our time together throughout the weekend included sharing a few meals and some funny stories about how frequently and horrendously people tend to butcher our names. Names like Fitz and Meb are apparently impossible for some. No, they're not as common as John and Jane, but come on! They're four and three letters each. Why many include an R in my name and call me Fritz, I'll never know. Saying "Meb" correctly seems pretty easy to me too.

I was also able to turn my microphone over to him a couple of times at our start lines so he could share some motivation with our athletes. They loved him. One of the things I appreciated most about Meb was his taste in friends. He and I both flocked to our driver, Joe Bryan, who works for the City of Philadelphia. Joe's laid back, hard-working, considerate, and fairly unimpressed by "famous running people." Like me, he just prefers good people. Joe offered to drive to the end of the earth to get Meb a Philly Cheesesteak and me some chocolate-covered strawberries.

That night I also spent time with a pack of fanatical runners known as the *Boston Buddies*. These are serious marathoners who are passionate about training for, qualifying for, and conquering the Boston Marathon. This year, a few dozen of them came to Philly to support the AACR. I met one of their most vocal athletes, Marty Clark, at the party and knew we'd likely go on to become friends for life. Marty is high energy and bursts with joy like I do, so our connection was immediate. Here's the cool part. As we walked past each other near the buffet, Marty stopped me to tell me that he loved my hair. Now, it was blissful for me to both have hair and to have someone compliment me on it. But the neatest part was that Marty was a professional hair stylist! For some reason, Marty's opinion mattered more because he was a pro.

November 22. Friday.

After participating in a ceremonial ribbon cutting at noon to open the expo, I made a beeline for my stage so I could set up for my scheduled presentation. A little more than half of my presentations are designed around helping people improve their health or their performance as an athlete. The others are designed almost purely for entertainment. This one was the latter. *Race Fails, Fun and Motivation* is based around my absolute worst, most frustrating, and ludicrous race experience ever. The number of things that went completely wrong between the start and finish of that half-marathon, combined with the absolute insanity of certain situations, just leaves my audiences in stitches. I can't tell you any more, but if you'd like to hear the rest, I guess you'll have to attend one of my presentations. Personally, I enjoy *Race Fails* because my audience's responses are so rewarding. They gasp, squirm in their seats, and belly laugh all the way through. Besides sharing my own freakish experience, I share many stories that my running friends have shared with me. I believe this particular presentation is such a home run because my audiences can completely identify with shit hitting the fan on race day. Another wonderful thing about *Race Fails* is that new material is constantly being produced! Is running hard? Sure! Is it also sometimes hilarious? Definitely.

This stage was set up in the dead center of the packed venue with lines of chairs in front of it and zero walls surrounding it. This type of layout can be difficult as it often leads to both presenters and audience members becoming distracted. On the bright side, it also lends itself to extra people dropping into an audience because they were captivated while walking by. The setup seemed to work in my favor because I was able to stay focused and continuously draw people in. As usual, my attendees and I shared an enormous amount of laughs, and a bunch of folks stayed after to meet, take pics, and share their own funny running experiences. As a newcomer to this event, I was already making myself at home and finding my groove.

When I left the expo, I took the opportunity to do more sightseeing. I was already heading toward our start and finish line area to pick up my announcer book, which had all of the schedules and sponsor blurbs, so I decided to see the things in the vicinity. First up, it was my chance to say, "Yo, Adrian. I did it!" Yes, the famous Rocky Balboa statue sits at the base of the Philadelphia Museum, and his footprints reside at the top of the steps leading up to it. The museum is the first thing our runners stride by after they pass the start line. After posing for a pic with the Rocky statue in the obligatory pose with my fists raised up toward the sky, I decided to check out the museum.

I spent a few enthralling hours inside of it and left with several observations. First, it's gargantuan. The interior space is 633,825 square feet and trudging through just half of it was exhausting. I arrived in Philadelphia feeling pretty decent, but if I had stuck it out to explore every nook and cranny of that behemoth, I would have been whacked. Second, it truly is the keeper of some mesmerizing artwork. I saw pieces from Picasso, Rembrandt, Monet and all of the other art world titans. The collections were wildly diverse and there was definitely something for everyone. There were paintings, sculptures, furniture, textiles, photographs and more. Lastly, it was worth every penny. I think I dropped about $20-$25 to go in, and I'd happily do it again. That place is an American treasure. After grabbing some Mexican takeout for dinner, I was pleased to return to my hotel before 8 p.m. to rest up for Saturday's races.

November 23. Saturday.

I felt like a kid at Christmas as I leapt into my Uber, headed to the start line. I was more than stoked to be announcing this mega-sized event and the 30-degree temps weren't going to keep me down. I had wisely invested time and energy into researching some cold-weather gear, knowing that Philly in the fall could be frigid. I almost always tend to go wrong in the pants department at races, but was guided by some northern gals to buy a pair of fleece-lined lululemon tights. Boy, was I glad I did. They were skinny like regular tights, but they actually kept me warm. I consider them one of the mysteries of the universe. I was also gifted with an official Philadelphia Marathon staff parka, which was designed specifically for cold, wet weather. Lastly, I bought a case, yes a case, of those magical hand warmers, which I had generously distributed inside my clothes, and across my body.

Speaking of clothing, our athletes showed up dressed in their finest garbage bags with strategic holes cut out for their heads and arms, and their most adorable throw-away clothes. What the hell am I talking about, you ask? Well, it's a long-standing tradition for runners to dress like vagrants at marquee running events. I'm kidding. Runners have to manage their body temperature changes wisely. If they show up to an event on a cold morning and stand around for an hour or so before the start of their race, they need to bundle up to stay warm. But, as soon as they start running they'll start to sweat, so they're likely going to want to disrobe a bit as their core temperature increases. To avoid ditching their pricey jacket or having to wrap a favorite hoodie around their waist, they wear something dirt cheap or something they simply don't care about leaving behind. Some people will even go thrift shopping to purchase something disposable. Right before athletes cross the start line, you'll see them throwing weird garments in the air as they run. From my vantage point on stage, it's a silly fashion show that I enjoy commenting on. Everyone gets a few chuckles out of it, and all discarded items are usually donated to a worthy cause.

Almost 15,000 athletes lined up for the 7:30 a.m. start of the Dietz and Watson Half Marathon. Their energy was kinetic, and I absorbed every iota of it. They were receptive to my jokes, responsive when I asked them questions, and eager to shout and celebrate on cue. To be honest, the crowd was so large that I could only see the first half of them from my start line stage. Most importantly though, I could hear them, and they could hear me. On top of giving instructions and making sure everyone had a memorable experience, there were some scripted moments to pilot, which included recognizing our sponsors. Of course, that began with the half marathon title sponsor, Dietz and Watson, who had an executive on hand to say a few words. I also had Mitch Stoller, Executive

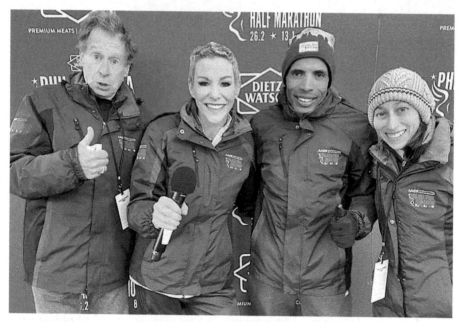

With running royalty. Bill Rodgers, Meb Keflezighi and Desiree Linden.

Director of the AACR at my side, to greet the crowd. This was when I took the opportunity to do exactly what I was hired to do. Make an impact on the masses and a compelling case for joining the AACR's Team Runners for Research.

I wasn't completely bald anymore, but my hair still told a poignant story, so I removed my fuzzy hat, lowered the music, and asked for the crowd's full attention. While I live for the roar of the crowd, it's also pretty cool to have the power to temporarily silence one. I started by asking if anyone in the crowd had ever lost someone they loved or had been affected by cancer. Almost 100% of our runner's hands went up in the air. And that's when I told them that I had been too. In fact, for almost a year, I had been battling breast cancer with chemotherapy, surgery, and radiation. My year had been difficult, but thanks to the AACR, those who fund research, do research, and implement quality research, there was a light at the end of the tunnel for me. I then asked if anyone in the crowd planned to come back to run during the Philadelphia Marathon weekend the following year, which yielded a huge response. Then I told them that they could help fight cancers of all kinds by agreeing to join

Team Runners for Research when they registered for 2020. It was free to do, would come with significant benefits (free shirt, VIP tent access, extra medal), and they could follow their hearts if they wanted to fundraise. I then asked the crowd if they would join our team in 2020 and the response was practically deafening.

While the AACR's name was on all of the Philadelphia Marathon promotional material, the web site, shirts, and more … I bet up until that point, many within this running community had no idea what it was all about. While I would never in a trillion years volunteer to go through the hell I've endured because of breast cancer, I do appreciate some of the power that I've been able to wield because of it. I'm a passionate professional who has always been motivated to help others live better and longer. It's who I am and what I do. I enjoy compelling people to do their annual exams, squeeze their stuff, and fundraise to find cures. Getting a crowd 15,000-strong to laser focus on the AACR and fundraising for cancer research for even just a few minutes that morning meant something extraordinarily special to me. It will lead to more action, dollars, and cures for sure.

My new friend, Keturah Duncan, belted out the national anthem in her rich and soulful voice. Then it was time to yell, "Runners, set, go!" My custom-mixed start music blended the first few bars of the Rocky theme song into a zipped up version of Elton John's Philadelphia Freedom. By the time we launched that first wave, our athletes were jumping up and down raring to go. It was precisely the type of organized mayhem I strive for at my start lines and, man, did I enjoy the hell out of it. When my athletes are energized like that, I just about burst at the seams. It's kismet. I have no idea how many corrals we started because I lost track. But, what I can tell you is, it was a party from beginning to end.

I had about one hour at the half marathon finish line before I had to go back and start the Rothman Orthopaedics 8K. Even though many of our athletes had already run the half marathon that morning, they were all bursting at the seams again. One of the things I thoroughly enjoyed about the start of the 8K is that our athletes made a quick u-turn about a tenth of a mile after they crossed the start line, forcing them to run past me a second time. Holy moly, this was fun. Do you know how kids enthusiastically wave at their parents every single time they make eye contact while doing circles on a merry-go-round? That's exactly what it felt like. I was the race mommy with her 5,000-plus children on the course. As they ran by me after their u-turn, they waved, danced and pointed at their shirts, hoping that I would boldly recognize their team names or the charitable organizations they were running for. And I was happy to do so. If I haven't said it before, my profession doesn't suck.

When it was time to officially leave the start line I was pretty bummed. The only saving grace was that I was returning to the finish line, which was almost as fun. One thing on the agenda that was totally odd for me was promoting hot dog consumption. Our half marathon title sponsor Dietz and Watson had a clever campaign taking place. For every free hot dog eaten at the finish line festival, they would donate one dollar to the AACR. I was happy to plug the opportunity, and I did so frequently. But as a fitness expert it was the first time in my life I'd promoted hot dogs!

As the half marathon wound down, I hustled out to get to my 1 p.m. presentation at the expo. I had a little less than an hour to take an Uber to the hotel, run upstairs to grab my laptop, and walk a few blocks to the expo. While I should have been able to do all of this and arrive at my presentation with about 20 minutes to spare, things did not go my way. Due to the races, many of the roads were closed, so my Uber took forever to pick me up, and didn't drop me off until 12:50 p.m. Can you imagine how desperate I was to be on time? It's one thing to be late for an appointment or a meeting. It's a far more heinous infraction to be late for an *audience.* Never in my entire life have I been late to my own speaking engagement, and I wasn't going to let this be the day. Once I escaped my Uber, I sprinted past the doorman, through the hotel lounge and lobby, which was way larger than it had to be. This wasn't a little hotel. This was one of those fancy big-city types that wow you as you enter. I must have taken 300 steps before I reached what seemed to be the slowest elevators on the planet. After I landed on the 25th floor, which might as well have been located on the moon, I ran down the annoyingly long hallway to my room. Why are my hotel rooms always at the very end of the hallway? Perhaps hotels don't want to centrally locate their noisiest guest? Anyway. I threw my laptop into my backpack and sprinted back to the elevator, with said laptop bouncing heavily on my back. Then I raced out of the hotel and ran several blocks to the convention center, all while weaving through and around hordes of people on the sidewalks. I felt like a total badass when I climbed onto my stage at 1 p.m. on the dot. It was intense. And, for a girl who was still trying to manage the side effects of chemo, it was even more impressive. I'm pretty sure Usain Bolt would have given me some sort of slow clap for this one.

I took several deep breaths to recover from my million-yard dash, while at the same time plugging my laptop into the audio/visual system and clipping the lavalier microphone to my shirt. I greeted my audience while explaining my frantic race to get to them; they seemed to be entertained by my harried experience. And because I ended up being punctual, I had a good laugh at myself too.

For the first time, I was presenting *My Noisy Cancer Comeback*. Sound familiar? Since the AACR specifically hired me because of the impact I could have on their behalf, I thought it would make sense to dedicate one of my presentations to my breast cancer battle. I normally do not utilize PowerPoint presentations when I speak, but I had worked diligently on a photo-centric slideshow to help me share my experience more vividly. My mission was to tell my story (an abridged version of this book) in a reasonably upbeat and funny way. I also shared some of the hard truths and difficult moments, but I kept things light and focused on the laughs.

"The best-laid plans of mice and men often go awry." Famed poet Robert Burns nailed it! While the start of my story detailing my diagnosis was pretty easy to get through, I hit a roadblock around slide number nine. I had included a 60-second video of me choking back tears while talking about my hair falling out. I included it because it was real, raw, and enlightening. I hit "play" to start the video and watched the audience as they took the clip in. I was taken back as a handful of people began to cry and many others looked horrified. Oh, how I wished I could have taken it back and erased their sadness. Bringing people down was not my intention at all. I was just trying to share the intensity of my moment and situation. I was rattled. I've spent decades helping people learn while laughing and I've never induced tears. I felt terrible that I'd made them feel bad, and there was nothing I could do to undo it. So, I did the only thing I could do. I forged on with the next slide and the next story. I dug deep to add levity, but the entire thing felt like a roller coaster. Highs, lows, deep lows, and some more highs.

While the feedback to my presentation was outstanding, it has taken me some time to wrap my head around it. Much like within the pages of this book, talking about my experiences with breast cancer cannot be all rainbows and puppy dogs. I still feel 100% confident that keeping my hardships to myself as I was going through them was the right decision for me. I would have despised public discussions about my illness, pain, suffering, and stress. And I would have loathed the pity too. But now I strongly feel that sharing my experiences moving forward is a powerful tool for awareness and early detection. I suppose I'm just going to have to get used to it.

After I wrapped things up, I was greeted with tons of hugs, love, and kindness from my audience. The audience was a mix of old friends and new ones. A true highlight of the weekend transpired when I reunited with my sweet pal, 10-year-old Emily Keicher. I've welcomed Emily through the finish lines of the Buffalo Marathon Kid Races and the 5K several times, and she always makes my heart explode. She is smart, funny, sunshiny, determined, beautiful, and oh yeah ... she has spina bifida. The sweet girl is an adaptive runner who uses support braces and a killer bright pink sports chair to help her go the distance. Emily's can-do spirit and megawatt smile are infectious, so I was grateful to see her. There couldn't have been a more perfect reason for me to get out of my own head, relax, and just enjoy some quality time with one of my littlest heroes.

November 24. Sunday.

Once again, I sprang out of bed, eager to get to the start line. Sure, it was only 4 a.m., but I was meeting almost 13,000 athletes this morning and was chomping at the bit to get to them. I bundled up in as many layers as I could and stuffed hand warmers into wherever they would fit. The day was projected to be brutally cold, and this very lean Floridian was preparing to battle Mother Nature. I've never been good with cold temperatures, but if I was given the opportunity to announce a race in Antarctica, I'd take it. The Philly weather wasn't going to deter me. After another Uber ride to the start line, it was go-time. This was the perfect prototypical northeastern race. We were in the heart of an iconic American city, surrounded by famous landmarks, and it was absolutely frigid, with pouring rain and gray skies. This setting simply doesn't exist in the south. I was shaking in my boots and parka, but I was also loving every minute of it.

As I've noted before, I'm obsessed with gargantuan crowds. The more, the merrier is an understatement. Here's a little secret: Getting 10 people pumped up and rowdy can be awkward. Why? Because everyone feels like they're on display, and people in small groups often don't want to stand out. But in large crowds, the kind I typically get to work with, people tend to feel well-hidden and liberated. Combine big numbers with brisk temps and electrifying music, and my start lines look almost as wild as a mosh pit. Once we were done with the scripted pre-race rigmarole and the dignitary speeches, it was time to bring down the house.

The music blared like a rock concert, and when I told our athletes there were only 60 seconds until the start of the first corral, they nearly lost their minds. Since our elite runners were jumping up and down to stay warm, I bellowed, "Philadelphia. It's time for jumpiiiiiing!" And they all did. Have you ever seen 13,000 people jumping up and down? It was mind-blowing fun. In fact, I was jumping too (and praying I wouldn't bring down the entire stage). Moments like these are why I love what I do. More precisely, they're why every single time I boarded a plane sick as hell, it was worth it. Getting to play ringleader for the greatest athletic shows on earth is a gift I will never, and I do mean never, willingly surrender. Each athlete, smile, hoot, holler, jump, and step they take fuels me. Every single one of the extraordinary people I host feeds my soul.

One funny experience I had at the start line came as a result of a bit of airhorn confusion. For the record, I do not like air horns. They come across as low budget and remind me of teeny little 5K races. And while I love teeny 5K races and participate in them often, a big race with a professional announcer should utilize that announcer's big voice or something better, like a cannon. However, things tend to go awry when you encourage or allow dignitaries and special guests to honk that air horn. It's kind of fun and makes them feel important. On this particular day, though, none of our guests could get the timing right. When done properly, you should hear, "Runners, Seeeeet..." and then the air horn gets blown in the place of the word "GO." Unfortunately, eighty percent of our guests screwed up and blew the horn as I yelled "set." One of the guests was a really nice executive who was standing directly next to me. When it was his turn to use the horn, he pointed it directly at my head and blasted it straight into my ear. If I hadn't seen it coming, rotated, and leaned back a bit, he would have blown out my eardrum for sure.

Throughout the hour of pre-race announcements and the 20-30 exciting minutes of race starts, the rain continuously pelted us in the face. Our athletes deserved so much credit. Their 26.2-mile journey hadn't even begun, and they were already frozen and soggy. Running a race can be tricky. You often have to overcome so many obstacles that have nothing to do with whether or not your body is prepared to go the distance. Weather, wardrobe, hydration, nutrition, and potholes can either make or break you. I was impressed as hell that they showed up and were ready to blast off, despite the weather. Once everyone crossed the start line and began their trek, I headed over to the finish line, which was only a 5-minute walk away. The finish line stage was equipped with a canopy cover, which proved to be a godsend on that very wet day. Since spectators hadn't arrived yet, I was more than happy to dethaw and grab some breakfast in the heated VIP tent.

The tent was filled with muckety-mucks who were in search of the same things I was: warmth and food. I plopped down at a table with my hot tea and thoroughly enjoyed chatting with Desiree Linden (Des for short), the 2018 Boston Marathon champion. I told Des how much I loved the look of intensity she wore as she earned her title in similarly cold, wet weather. If you've not seen it, just search online for video footage of her running that race. You'll see the look I'm talking about. I laughed when she told me that she was glad I thought she looked determined because, in reality, she was scared. "I was terrified," she said. That was a pretty honest thing for her to reveal, and I loved it. We talked a bit more about pace, mean girls, and our experiences in the industry. She was delightful, and I thoroughly enjoyed our little chunk of girl talk.

I spent the next seven hours celebrating and congratulating our athletes at the finish line, which was a pleasure, despite the dank

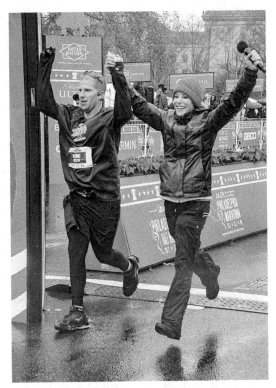

Running Marc Kassel across his Philadelphia Marathon finish line. Photo by Island Photo

conditions. Yes, I trembled nonstop, but I couldn't complain because our runners were experiencing something much worse. After all, it was snowing and sleeting at various locations on the course. So, while I wasn't comfortable, I was in way better shape than they were. About five hours after I launched the marathon, I went down to greet finishers and wait for my new sightseeing buddy, Marc Kassel. I wanted to greet him and personally run him through the finish line.

I went down a bit prematurely and ended up waiting in the cold pouring rain for 20 minutes or so. Eventually, I saw Marc approaching, and our spectators went bonkers when I told them about his recent 100+ pound weight loss. When Marc got to me (about 5 yards in front of the finish line), he hugged me and couldn't let go. The man was frozen solid and violently shaking. He was completely soaked and looked as if he'd just climbed out of a pool. The freezing temperatures combined with the rain, sleet, and snow mixed like oil and water. Not well. I was insanely proud and amazed that he'd crushed all three races that weekend, but I was also kind of worried for him. I thought, "Bless his heart! He needs to warm up." So, I pried his arms off of me and got him to move again so we could cross the finish line together.

After I put the finisher medal around his neck, I brought him over to my stage security to ask for help. I was the new girl in town, so I asked extra nicely. I said, "I haven't asked for any extras at all this weekend, but it would mean a lot to me if my friend could come into the VIP tent to warm up." Thankfully, security had no problem with that. When I came in to grab some hot tea a while later, I found him in the tent, surrounded by people trying to help him. Eventually, he was able to change his clothes and hobble back to his hotel. I had nothing but respect for Marc and everyone else who ran that race.

Monday morning I left the AACR Philadelphia Marathon, flying high and feeling proud that I'd added this quality event to my calendar. I also left further motivated to continue speaking out for cancer causes. There was power in my platform, and people responded to me. While I had no interest in wearing ribbons, I had a ton of interest in compelling people to get their annual exams and do their own self-exams. I was also eager to support efforts to fund more research. The more I spoke about cancer, the more necessary I believed it was to continue speaking, and writing, about cancer. In fact, since you're almost at the end of my book, it's a good time to ask.

Have you done a self-exam since you started reading it? Have you squeezed your stuff? Groped your boobs or squished your testicles? Have you made an appointment for an annual exam you may not have without my influence? If the answer is yes, then you've proved my point. If telling this story and talking about squeezing stuff gets people to do better and be better, then I'm successfully continuing on with my professional mission to help others live better and longer. If you haven't squeezed your stuff, then WHAT THE HELL ARE YOU WAITING FOR? Put your hand under your shirt or in your pants and have a feel. It's your hand

and your stuff! No one else has the same right and responsibility to your body that you do, so get on with it. I hope you find nothing, but if you do, I hope you pick up the phone and call your doctor immediately. Not after you speak to a friend or family member. Not after you query Google. Just call your damn doctor.

November 26. Tuesday.

My insane life as a human yo-yo continued, and I was back in the chemo chair for round #13. The contrasting image of me 48 hours earlier standing on a brightly lit stage at the helm of a jumping mob of athletes was still puzzling. One of the niceties of the day, though, was a complimentary housecleaning visit from a local company — A Personal Elf. Through their partnership with the American Cancer Society, they had donated two 2-hour visits to my home. Rob had been doing everything he could to keep up with our house, but he was also working and daddying full time, so certain things needed a little more attention. My "Elves" gave my bathrooms a solid scrubbing and cleaned my kitchen floors. I can't tell you how refreshing it felt to have these important chores done for us. While cancer has wielded some nasty byproducts, this is the perfect example of the goodness I experienced because of it.

I've mentioned chemo brain quite a few times, but haven't described it fully. For me, it manifested in ways that made me appear and feel like a total airhead. Have you ever walked into your kitchen, opened the fridge, and wondered, "What the hell am I in here looking for?" That's been me on countless occasions. I didn't forget the big things: people, places, or major concepts. But I struggled to remember other details such as friends' names, minor obligations, and conversations I'd already had. I was constantly asking and re-asking my kids the same questions about school. "I've already told you that, Mom!" they would say. Sometimes they'd show aggravation toward me, and other times they'd just laugh. I was constantly apologizing and asking them to humor me and re-answer the redundant questions. But Ginger and Parker weren't the only victims of my repeat conversations. I also frequently forgot to return calls or messages, which made me look like a jerk on more than 5,000 occasions. And worst of all, sometimes I'd forget whether or not I'd taken my prescription drugs each morning and night. I eventually bought a pill organizer that made me feel like I was 97 years-old. I felt like a dork depending on the little box with dose compartments, but I couldn't risk not taking my prescriptions or doubling the dosage. Lastly, I have also forgotten a bunch of memories. People have brought up things we've done together and I haven't had a clue what they were talking about. Sometimes I feel that my sharpness will return along with my short-term memory. However, other times I'm semi-concerned that I may have lost some of the long term memories forever.

Fitzness Log

This is the month I got smart and switched things up a bit. Instead of scheduling chemo for 9 a.m. like I had been doing all year, I pushed my infusions back to lunchtime. This allowed me to go to the gym and get a killer workout in before I got pumped full of things that made me tired and loopy. Even though I still didn't look forward to infusion days, I felt extremely empowered starting things off with a swim and some strength training.

The other thing I had to address was my chemo butt. What is chemo butt, you ask? Well, I'll tell you. After Godzilla made those 12 pounds fall off, I looked in the mirror and was shocked to find that my juicy booty was no more. All of the junk in my trunk had disappeared and I was left with a very disappointing, flat-like-a-pancake, chemo butt. Now, my pre-cancer tush was not the type any dignified rapper would ever write lyrics about. However, it was pretty decent for a girl my size. Was it small? Yes. Was it firm, round and perky? Definitely! So my mission was to earn it back. Lunges, step-ups, squats, and monster walks became my go-to for fixing chemo butt.

Chapter 12

Aren't I Lucky to Have Survived So Much Bad Luck?

December 7. Saturday.

This was my second year announcing the Savannah Bridge Run 5K and 10K. I was stoked to have Parker and his BFF, Kayla, accompany me to this charming city, which is only a three-hour drive from home. While Savannah is unique in so many ways, crossing the Talmadge Bridge is an absolute treat and makes these races quite popular. Our 5K runners cross it once. Our 10K runners cross it twice. Runners who do both races, AKA the Double Pump Challenge, get to cross it three times. How neat is that?

The beginning of my day was far too exhilarating. My first start in the morning was for the 5K and I launched that race from the other side of the bridge. What's the other side you ask? Well, this race has three different staging areas. Two start lines and one finish line. The finish line and the start of the 10K are both seated in Downtown Savannah. This is our home base. Since the 5K race starts across the bridge on Hutchinson Island, that's referred to as the other side. This meant that I had to yell "GO" to launch the 5K on Hutchinson Island, and then get to the finish line in Downtown Savannah before the runners did to welcome them.

In order to make this happen, I had to throw on my backpack and leave the stage I'd been using for pre-race announcements as soon as the anthem finished. With my wireless microphone in hand, I'd walk about 10 yards in front of our start line and get folks pumped up from there. Once the clock struck 8 a.m., I would yell "GO" and then jump into the open hatch of the pace car waiting right behind me. The pace car would then drive the course with our lead athletes following behind. As we approached the finish line, the pace car would speed up and then I'd bound out of the car, run 30 yards down the

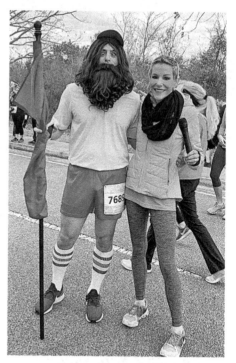

Run, Forrest, Run!

finish line chute, grab the microphone awaiting me, and boldly welcome our champion with the grandiosity that he deserved. Sounds easy enough, right? Wrong.

"Aren't I lucky to have survived so much bad luck?" is a quote from author Ashleigh Brilliant, and I think it fits the mood of that day perfectly. As I stood in front of the 5K start line, I could actually see the hunger on our runner's faces. They were either running to win or to at least set a PR. When the clock struck 8 a.m., I was yelling "Runners, set, goooo!" and running backward before I jumped into the hatch of the pace car, backside first. Unfortunately, I did not stick the way we had planned. In fact, I did not stick at all. Instead, I slid straight out of the slowly moving car. Thankfully, my feet hit the ground first, and I was able to keep my upper back in the car while running upside-down and backward to keep up with it. That was the good news. The bad news was that thousands of runners were barreling down on me as I dangled out of the back of that car. As my feet shuffled to keep up, all I could think about was how pathetic the news report was going to be about the cancer-stricken announcer lady who slipped out of a pace car and was trampled to her death by a pack of runners. I also thought about how viral the video would go if someone was recording this catastrophe. While I was shuffling for my life, our driver had absolutely no clue what was going on. I think I was able to squeak out the word "wait" at some point, but there was zero value to it because he couldn't hear me at all. After about 30 seconds, the photographer who was also in the back of the car grabbed me and yanked me in properly. Good grief! That was a close one. It took a few minutes for the shock to wear off, but I was quickly able to laugh off my blunder.

The rest of the plan went well, and I was able to beat our champion to the finish line. But our spectators were very confused when they saw me running down the finish line chute. Since I was the first person they saw and, because I was sprinting, they cheered wildly believing I was winning the race. I tried to wave off their applause, but I couldn't make them understand until I got on the microphone. I thought my drama for the day was complete when one of our race volunteers approached me with a smile and said, "Wow! You have so much blood on your face!" I replied with a curious, "What? What are you talking about?" Again, with a huge grin on her face, she said, "Your left cheek is covered with blood!" *Umm. Okaay.* Why she looked so happy about this I'll never know, but I put the microphone to my mouth and asked if I could get a paramedic to the tent. While I continued to welcome athletes, about four of our medics came over to check me out. There was blood. And lots of it. Fortunately, it was only a superficial cut high up on my left cheek. Chemo made my blood very thin, so it didn't take much to make me look like I'd been involved in a massacre. On a sadder note, gobs of blood had gotten all over my new yellow lululemon jacket. That was an expensive realization.

The rest of the day did not include any more llama drama. I started the 10K on flat land and enjoyed the finish line show as thousands of runners poured in. Many of them were dressed up for the post-race costume contest, which meant we had some athletic cupcakes, burglars, Santas, Whos from Whoville, superheroes, football players, and at least two Forrest Gumps. Mr. Gump appears at many of my races around the country, but since the famous park bench scene from the movie was filmed in Savannah's Chippewa Square, he always attends the Savannah Bridge Run.

December 25. Wednesday.

Sitting around the Christmas tree with Rob, the kids, and Piper felt extra special this year. As the magic of Santa faded away for Ginger and Parker, so had my affinity for all of the work that comes along with this holiday. Putting the tree up, decorating the house, shopping until I drop, and wrapping a gazillion gifts (yes, we go appallingly overboard) had become a bit tedious over the past few years. But not this year. Even with chemo #14 thrown in on December 16th, I felt grateful to be alive for another Christmas. I had fun buying our 10-foot tree at the Home Depot, turned on festive music, and forced the kids to look jolly as we decorated the tree. I even took the time to smile big while wrapping all of the presents. It's not that I operated like *The Grinch* in the past, but it's easy to become pretty aggravated with the mountain of work and effort that comes along with this holiday. When I thought back to how my year *might* have ended had I not found my lump when I did, I was pretty freaking giddy to be doing another Noel.

Most of our gifts were a big success, and we spent the afternoon at Rob's parents' house with his family from New Jersey. Since my diagnosis, his mom had volunteered to host all of the holidays, which took a lot off of our plates. Many years ago, she went through chemo herself, so she's been extremely concerned, considerate, and helpful throughout my treatment.

After Christmas dinner, we played all sorts of snarky board games, which led to hilarious conversations. We don't get to spend much time with our New Jersey peeps, so it was fun to hear so much from my niece Abby and her younger brothers Jack and Toby. I was a bit tired and queasy that night, but it didn't take away from my enjoyment of our company. Just being a part of Christmas and celebrating with loved ones was a genuine gift —and my most prized gift by far.

Fitzness Log

This month I switched from the warm pool to the lap pool and started actually swimming. Man, did that feel fantastic! Lap swimming is challenging and I loved getting my heart rate up. In fact, every time I paused at either end of the pool, huffing and puffing to catch my breath, I rejoiced. I started by tackling 10 minutes of laps every other day after my strength training and progressed by tacking on a few minutes of swimming whenever I could. I hadn't had a killer cardio workout since the beginning of the year and I was so happy to be on the comeback physically.

My eating habits still weren't very diverse. I was still gobbling up tangerines and guacamole like it was my job. But I was also trying to squeeze in any extra calories I could. You may be disappointed to read this, but French fries made their way into my mouth a few times a week. Sorry, not sorry.

Chapter 13

Small, But Mighty

January 1, 2020. Wednesday.

Happy New Year! After watching the ball drop on television, I was excited to leave 2019 in the dust. I was ready to move into a new year with much more health and energy on the agenda. I had conquered a million things in 2019, including saving my life, but it was definitely the worst year ever. Sure, I still had eight more rounds of Godzilla to go, but they had no chance of wrecking me in the same way my 2019 treatments had. I was, however, going to start a new oral drug called Tamoxifen. I would take it every single night for 10 years. I chose to start on January 1, 2020, so I could officially stop on January 1, 2030. It would make such a nice round number. In short form, Tamoxifen is given to people diagnosed with hormone-receptor-positive breast cancer to reduce the risk of cancer coming back. Since my diagnosis, I've heard women complain about their side effects from Tamoxifen. Some of these include joint pain, weight gain, hot flashes, mood swings, and more. I've also heard that the side effects come on almost instantly. Not really uplifting, huh? However, I've already been taking it for six months and I've had zero adverse reactions. Because Tamoxifen is a powerful tool for preventing a recurrence, I'm thrilled to be one of the lucky girls who isn't being punished for using it.

On the professional front, I was irrationally excited about the year that laid ahead. My race announcing calendar was filled to the brim and I couldn't wait to saturate my life with happy, healthy people. I was booked almost every weekend of the spring, summer, and fall. Plus, I planned to feel healthy and strong for all of them. What could be better?

January 18. Saturday.

I was thrilled to be back in California and standing on a stage next to Rudy. Team Noisy was back for the Carlsbad Marathon, which we've announced together for years. We were kicking the weekend off with our Kids Marathon Mile at Legoland. Thousands of kids and their parents lined up for seven different starts, and the fact that we got to be their support crew couldn't be cooler. As usual, Rudy an-

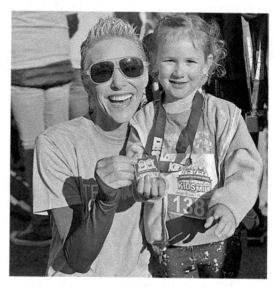

Julia Shaver made my day. I love this little one.

nounced the finish line and I took care of the start. After notifying the parents that none of them were at risk of stepping on Legos, we were set for shenanigans. Of course, we had the mommy, daddy, and family dance parties, we shouted for our favorite Lego sets (Star Wars® being the decisive winner), and jumped up and down before I yelled, "GO." These families were eager to have a blast and went along with all of my silliness.

One very special runner showed up just to see me, something I hope she'll continue to do for the rest of her life. Julia Shaver, 4, stole my heart two years prior at the 2017 Carlsbad Marathon Mile. I was up on my start line tower wearing a bright pink jacket, when she and her parents walked across the mostly empty parking lot toward the bib pickup area. As I was talking, the newly two-year-old Julia turned her head to see me, stopped dead in her tracks, ditched her parents, and ran straight toward me with a dazzling smile. I abandoned Rudy and bolted down the tower's stairs to meet this teeny toddler with the most adorable auburn ponytails jetting out of the sides of her head. As we came together, she reached her arms up to me for a big hug and I crouched down to give her one. It was possibly the sweetest moment of my career. Eventually, her parents, BreeAnn and Andy, got to both of us, and we all introduced ourselves. They were tickled by my instant connection with their daughter. I poured major praise over Julia as she finished her first race ever, and our love fest continued the next day during the big races. Her daddy was running the half marathon, and she came out with mommy to cheer him on. As I walked down the finish line chute of our Surf Sun Run 5K to greet our athletes, I found that little cutie pie with her arms stretched out for me again. I got to walk around with Julia in my arms for a bit, which made all of the sweet stuff squish out of my heart. It was then that BreeAnn told me that Julia hadn't stopped talking about my long blonde hair and pink jacket since the previous night.

We soon connected via social media and have stayed in touch for years. Although they moved about an hour away from Carlsbad to Orange County, they let me know that they were coming back to see me and do the Legoland Marathon Mile. I couldn't wait to see Julia. She's a quiet little ladybug, but she greeted me with a warm hug and lots of sweetness. Her parents were kind and shared their concerns over my health. Mostly, our reunion was filled with amazement for how much Julia had grown and what it meant to me that they came out again. I'm hoping she'll always return for our annual reunions.

After breakfast with a group of running friends, we jumped in Rudy's car and went to the race expo for a security meeting. It's pretty interesting to hear about all of the measures taken by different agencies to protect us all on race day. I'm not going to describe them in detail, but they sure are reassuring. Once we were done talking safety, we headed into the expo to check out the vendors and visit with some athletes. You know how sometimes the right person comes into our lives at the right time? Beth Kent was that person for me. She lives in Fort Lauderdale, where I grew up, but we'd never met outside of social media. For some reason, Beth decided that she had to run a Team Noisy race and flew all the way across the country to run the Carlsbad Half Marathon. Pretty incredible, right? Beth and I had been texting that day, so we would be able to catch each other at the expo. When we met. Beth exploded with positive energy. She overflowed with excitement about meeting us in person, and was dripping with genuine concern over me and my health. It was the type of worry you'd expect from your favorite aunt. She was a businesswoman and avid runner who regularly traveled for races. She also spoke a million miles a minute and laughed a lot, which made me instantaneously happy to be her friend. I think we hung out for 30 minutes before parting ways, but not before she handed both of us gifts.

I'm going to backtrack a bit here before I tell you what Beth gave me. For reference, I was really struggling with my weight loss. I was down to 112 pounds and had lost almost all of my curves. I used to be a size 3 or small. Now I was a size 0, 1, or extra small. None of my dresses fit, nor did many of my other clothes. Everything sagged or hung strangely on my stick-figure body. I could still pull off most of my fitness apparel, thank goodness, but even my running tights were a little loose. That was fairly unnerving. To top it off, the night before, I had gone into lululemon to do a little shopping at a location I had been in many times before. lululemon sizes are weird, and I normally wear a size 6 in their stuff. I wanted to buy things that would continue fitting once I was able to put some weight back on, so I was still looking for size 6. An employee soon came over to ask me what I was looking for and what size I wanted. When I responded, her eyes bugged out, and she said, "You are definitely not a size 6." I froze like a deer in headlights and my eyes welled up with tears. I knew my mom could see how thin I was, but the sassy lady in my head kept telling me that I looked normal to the general public. I was speechless. Thankfully, Rudy was with me and intervened. He ushered me away and told the employee to grab that size 6. When I was in the dressing room, he secretly gave her the scoop. I felt a little bit better after the retail therapy, but continuously adapting to my new appearance was complex. It was great to have hair again, and I'd been styling it into a very fun faux-hawk. But, sometimes, I just felt like I looked like a 12-year-old boy. Where did my glamorous long hair and curvy booty go?

Back to Beth's gift or should I say gifts. She gave me a heartfelt letter and a beautiful scarf, but what meant the most to me and brought the biggest smile to my face was a half-dollar sized silver medallion with the phrase "Small but Mighty" etched into it. How did she know? OMG! How in the freaking world did she know? Of course, she couldn't have known. She just happened to be the right person to come into my life at the right time. Was I small? Yep. Was I mighty? One hundred per-freak-ing-cent! I needed to remember that. Beth's presence and her present were a fabulous morale boost for me. And as far as the medallion goes, I keep it with my flight attendant's lucky rock. And whenever I struggle with my size, chemo-induced fatigue, or other temporary nonsense I try to remind myself that I *am* "Small but Mighty."

January 19. Sunday.

The Tri-City Medical Center Carlsbad Marathon, Half Marathon, and Surf Sun Run 5K might as well be renamed Rudy's Birthday Party. Sure, most of our athletes came out because they wanted to run in one of San Diego's most dazzling beachside cities. But it also seemed that a good chunk showed up just to bestow happy wishes onto my announcing partner. And he ate it all up. Before the start of the half-marathon, a few friends and organizers asked me to surprise Rudy by singing Happy Birthday to him. I wanted Rudy to feel special and enjoy all of the love he deserved, so I quickly agreed. Unfortunately, what we had hoped to be a massive singalong with our 5,000 athletes, turned into more of a pitchy Fitz solo. The way the start line was set up, most of our athletes were corralled behind a curve in the road. We couldn't really see or hear them, which didn't work out in my favor. I ended up having to carry the weight of the tune so it didn't just die out. That was awkward.

Thinking back to my experience singing the anthem at the Ruffalo Stampede in Buffalo when my iPad overheated, I couldn't help but wonder why for the second time in a year, I've had to publicly sing the two most difficult songs in American culture. It's not that I like to sing, but if I were to choose a song to sing publicly, it'd be something with a bit of zing like Garth Brooks' "Callin' Baton Rouge" or Aretha Franklin's "Respect." Basically songs I could compensate for with some spunk and funky moves. I would not pick the National Anthem nor the birthday song. They left me with no wiggle room.

Speaking of the anthem, things went awry with that as well. After we had already asked everyone to turn to the flag and stand at attention, we couldn't get the iPad to play our recorded version. Now it was Rudy's turn to perform. Without giving it a second thought, he brought the microphone to his mouth and started crooning "Oh say can you see." He did an outstanding job, but it took every ounce of restraint not to fall apart laughing. It dawned on me that cameras were likely pointed our way, so I should look professional. While Team Noisy is not likely to secure a record deal or win a Grammy, we would definitely qualify for the "Think Fast" award, or whatever award people get for being willing to throw themselves under the bus for the benefit of an event. Does that even exist?

Luckily, these were the final goofs of the day. The rest of our morning and afternoon was filled with nothing but revelry and happiness. Rudy continuously encouraged me to take breaks, and I continuously told him to stop telling me to do so. I was feeling fabulous, and we had far too many friends racing that day for me to risk missing any of their finishes. It was as if nothing had changed.

January 27. Monday.

Before I sat down for chemo #16, I had an appointment with Dr. Gordan. My stomach had settled down, and the majority of the other significant side effects had subsided, but I had one new issue causing me problems. Peripheral Neuropathy. If you're unfamiliar, it's defined as a disease or dysfunction of one or more peripheral nerves, typically causing numbness or weakness. Specifically, my toes and feet were tingling like crazy. This unpleasant feeling persisted during the day, but really escalated at night. This left me squirming and reaching down to squeeze my tootsies until I'd eventually pass out. I emailed Dr. Gordan about it and he referred me to get acupuncture and B vitamins as a management tool. Now he had a new plan. He wanted to reduce my dosage of Godzilla to 75% of what I'd been receiving. My knee jerk response was to decline his offer. I'd had my foot on the gas doing everything possible to kill my breast cancer and prevent a recurrence. I didn't want to have anything less than my original and ideal prescription required. Dr. Gordan told me that sometimes neuropathy can be permanent, and since I was so athletic, this could really put a damper on my quality of life. That was compelling enough. We agreed to do one more full dose of Godzilla, and if I continued to experience nerve pain, we'd reduce the dose before the next round. And that's exactly what we did. The tingling remained, and I relented. Seventy-five percent would eventually be good enough for me. As time passed, my nerves chilled out and the pain went away.

Fitzness Log

I'm proud to share that I was finally able to charge up killer hill! January brought other great accomplishments in fitness as well. Plumpness was returning to my rear, and I was swimming further than ever. Once I became comfortable swimming 10 minutes of laps, I bumped things up to 15 minutes, 20 and then 30. Once I hit 30 minutes of swimming, I started aiming for distance instead and conquered 1,500 yards. The idea of competing in a sprint triathlon over the summer was starting to swirl around in my mind. Not only was my body overjoyed by being able to move vigorously again, but my mind was also bursting with pride over my regained capabilities. And I was also stoked about my tush.

Chapter 14

Cancer Can Be Funny
#FlushTwice

February 15. Saturday.

Mud Girl, a women's obstacle course race at the Jacksonville Equestrian Center was not the largest event on my calendar, but it could easily qualify as my favorite. That's because my sweet Ginger Bean shared the stage with me. She had recently been hired by several of my races to fill in for me when I was double-booked, so I brought her with me to Mud Girl as a practice run. Unsurprisingly, I had to hold on for dear life. We were handed "Pink Army" crew shirts and pink tutus upon arrival, which instantly set the mood for silliness. A DJ showed up shortly after, and we turned our continuous start line into a non-stop dance party. Our ladies were stoked to get muddy on about 15 giant hot pink obstacles, which all had funny names. Mudbumps, Megapipes, Pinkranhas, Athena, Jaws, and Pink Cheese were some of the fun challenges that laid ahead. There was absolutely nothing serious about this race — by design — and we had free rein to be as animated as we wanted. Since obstacle course races require much smaller starting corrals, maybe 50 people in each, we ended up yelling "GO" every 10 minutes for five hours. We went back and forth between instructions and entertainment, and I couldn't have been prouder that my 17-year-old baby could hang with her mom.

From the second we said, "Good morning" until the time our final athletes finished, Ginger was a dynamo. Her confident ad-libbing in front of our crowds was spectacular, her energy could have fueled a small town, and her ability to make everyone laugh was ab-

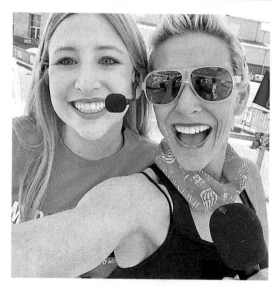

Ginger and I announcing Mud Girl. I couldn't have been prouder.

surd. Working together was a dream come true. The women were ultra playful and ate up our shenanigans, which made the time fly by. The fact that we were being compensated for having so much mother-daughter fun felt quasi-criminal. I knew that she would be fantastic as a race announcer, but she exceeded my expectations by far and those of the Mud Girl team too. In fact, a few hours into the event, our coordinator stopped by to show me a text he'd received from the Mud Girl owner, It read, "Fitz and Ginger are fantastic. Ginger is so fun, in 10 years, she'll be even better than her mom!" I beamed with pride.

The other highlight was that I was providing Ginger with a unique learning experience. And with that experience, an opportunity to earn a living. A "trade" you might call it. While I no longer felt like my life was in imminent danger, I still felt the urge to ingrain as much knowledge and capabilities in my kids as I could. She can make a decent living as a race announcer if she wants. It'll be her call, but I'm confident she now has a marketable skill.

February 21. Friday.

It's great to be a Florida Gator ... and a breast cancer survivor too! Never thought I'd be both, but there I was, down on the floor of the University of Florida's Stephen C. O'Connell Center waving and chomping at the crowds. This was the Gator "Link to Pink" Gymnastics meet, and I was the honored guest. Since gymnastics is a spring sport and doesn't compete in October during Breast Cancer Awareness Month, they picked their own date to raise awareness for breast cancer. A few weeks prior, I was asked to give a keynote speech after the meet for the other survivors and families in attendance. I was more than happy to take part.

I had been speaking about breast cancer around the country for a year, but all of my previous presentations had been to the masses. In those scenarios, I always spoke with the purpose of promoting prevention, early detection, and giving. While these themes were still relevant, this audience would definitely not need a lecture on getting mammograms. My task was then to figure out exactly what they did need.

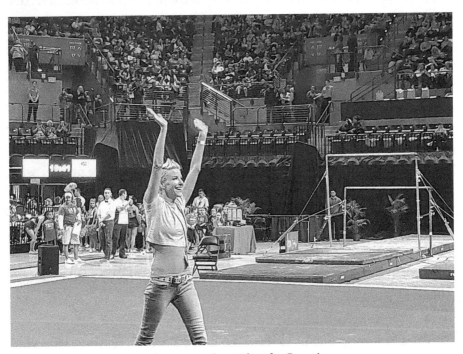

It's great to be a Florida Gator!

That's one of the secrets to being a successful speaker. Topics should always be geared precisely toward each audience. What does this specific group of people need to hear from me? If you know what it is and you can meet that need, then all you need is a game plan and a whole hell of a lot of charisma to captivate them. I decided what this particular group needed was to laugh. We all had this crappy disease in common, but as I've demonstrated in this book, some of those commonalities were actually quite comical. Perhaps an outsider couldn't pull off the jokes or funny stories, but I was going to endure chemo #17 four days before this presentation. I was scrawny and had spiky new hair. I had cancer street cred and a list of topics I thought everyone would get a kick out of.

Back to the beginning. UF welcomed about 100 breast cancer survivors, patients, and their families to the meet. They provided us all with complimentary seating, shirts, gifts, and a reception. I was given an extra perk: we were invited to sit down on the competition floor, alongside the athletic director, press, and emcee. Our seats were directly in front of the balance beam, which gave us an incredible view of all events. Ginger was occupied rehearsing for her role as Mae Peterson in her school performance of "Bye Bye Birdie," so Kayla came in her place. Being tagged as the honored guest of the evening meant that I would be introduced before the meet. While our sports announcer, Tom Collete, talked about who I was and what I did, I basically just stood out in the middle of the floor routine mat while chomping and waving. *If you have no idea what the heck "chomping" is, it's when Gators and Gator fans extend our arms straight out in front of us (right arm high, left arm low, creating a side V) and clap. Think about the soundtrack from the movie *JAWS* playing as thousands of people chomp with their arms. It's an iconic maneuver within college athletics that emulates the clashing teeth of a American alligator. There are very few universities, if any, with anything as identifiable. For the record, chomping is really fun and I love doing it.

As a Gator graduate twice over, I felt very loved when everyone cheered about me being a breast cancer survivor. I consider UF to be my second marriage and always enjoy being invited back to present or take part in school functions. This experience felt particularly warm and fuzzy. Once my individual introduction was complete, all of the other breast cancer patients and survivors joined me on the mat to welcome in our gymnasts. I laid my eyes on Cheryl Tyrone as she exited the massive pink inflatable Gator head tunnel everyone was entering through. I dashed over to steal a hug and join her. Again. I can't stand that any of my friends have had to deal with this crap, but it was cool to be with her doing something so fun. The crowd, decked out in free pink T-shirts UF provided, went bonkers for the large group of us. They also held up large signs with the names of those they've loved who've had breast cancer. The visuals were both impressive and meaningful. I was humbled and still mystified about being an official part of this group. Even with all of my treatments, I had felt like a breast cancer outsider. At least until that point. Then I was a certified member of the club no one wanted to be a part of. Club Breast Cancer! The good part: I had also made it into that exclusive squad of survivors.

The entire meet was very classy. The Florida Gators and their opponent, Alabama Crimson Tide, had chosen to ditch their traditional school colors in lieu of pink leotards. Team coaches, trainers, and support staff were also decked out in pink. And most of the crowd (about 10,000 people) was wearing pink. While I'm proud that my alma mater has gone to such lengths, you may be happy to know that many other universities make a similar effort. In fact, we've all seen football players take the field in pink socks, boxers in pink gloves, and tennis pros in pink tanks. According to the National Cancer Institute, besides non-melanoma skin cancers, breast cancer is the most common type of cancer diagnosis in the United States. It had 271,270 new cases in 2019, including mine. Everyone seems to know someone with it, love someone with it, or have lost someone with it. I certainly felt the embrace of all of those people in the O'Dome. And I hope the others in my club did too.

Once my Gators finished dominating the talented Crimson Tide, we went to the reception, which was held elsewhere in the arena. After snapping an adorable picture of Parker surrounded by The Dazzlers (members of the Gator dance team), we entered. The place was packed, and I took some time to check everyone out. While I didn't see many women much younger than myself (thank goodness), I did see all types of women. Literally. Women of every color. Women of all fitness levels. Women of various ages. Straight women. Gay women. Women of all religions and income levels. Breast cancer does not discriminate. This realization made me even more eager to get to the podium.

Within 10 minutes of my arrival, I was introduced by one of the Gator staff members and warmly welcomed by the audience. I started with my usual chemo brain disclaimer, just in case I lost any words along the way. Then I told a brief 60-second history of my year and followed that up with the fact that I'd decided to make fun of cancer. Or, at least the very absurd things I've experienced because of it. I won't describe it all, but I can tell you that the whole room burst into laughter when I told them about my flight attendant, the cookies, and the lucky rock. They also exploded with laughter over the bizarre order to "flush twice" for 48 hours after receiving chemo. Yes, we are all told to do this. No, almost nobody can justify why. As I went through my list of about 10 things I thought everyone would appreciate, the laughter became louder and lasted longer. It was such an uplifting time for us all. Even though I was the only person on the microphone, it felt like everyone was talking back through their laughter, nods, and hand motions. We were commiserating and finding the funny in this very serious disease. After thanking UF, the American Cancer Society, and the caregivers amongst us, it was time to go.

But before I left the podium, I thanked my fellow patients and survivors for being incredible role models. I told them how proud I was to stand with locked arms in such a strong group. And I meant it. As with my usual presentations, many of the women came over to meet me and chat. But this was unlike any of those other occasions because instead of me doling out extra pointers and advice, they were the ones sharing encouragement and guidance with me. Some stopped by to tell me that they were "X amount" years cancer-free, and one day, I'd be there too. Others shared recovery tips, and some just thanked me for making them laugh. I hit it off with a few new friends and we connected via social media shortly after.

It's no secret that I enjoy public speaking. Whether I'm teaching fitness, announcing races, or just providing entertainment, the one constant is that I'm connecting with large groups of people. My presentations regarding cancer have been extra rewarding. Partially because I have some important messages to share, but also because it's been fabulous to communicate about such a grim subject with so much joy. Sure, I've inserted some darker content into the mix, but I like that I can increase understanding of a very mean disease in a way that empowers people. I'm still not wearing ribbons, but I am forwarding the cause, and that makes me feel like I'm winning.

In the days leading up to this event, I was fretting over what to do if I was asked to wear a shirt with a pink ribbon on it. No, I didn't want to, but yes, I wanted to be a gracious participant. Is it a stupid dilemma? Perhaps! But at this point, I'm still not into it. Since it was my cancer, I get to react the way I want without feeling bad about it. I proactively chose to dress in a pretty pink shirt and push back the decision unless a request to change it arose. Guess what? It never did. I was given a gift bag with a shirt inside and I received no pressure to wear it. And when I got home, Ginger was more than excited to have a new shirt. What I've decided to do moving forward is just address each ribbon-wearing request as it comes. However, if you're reading this, please don't ask. I'll be happy to just wear pink. Pink's fabulous. It's a happy color to wear, and I feel pretty in it. If anyone needs proof that I'm a supporter of breast cancer research, I'll just show them my scars. I've got a handful of good ones!

Fitzness Log

My February workouts had been fantabulous and I was seriously contemplating a sprint triathlon over the summer. In fact, I'd made tentative plans to fly to Michigan after announcing the DC Wonder Woman Run series on June 28th to do Eva's Tri Goddess Triathlon on June 29th.

Her event entailed a quarter-mile swim, a 10.7-mile bike ride, and a 1.5-mile run. It was something to train for and look forward to. And it was a genius way to build athletic adventure back into my life. I was giddy. Since triathlons include running and biking, I was going to have to start putting effort into those activities as well. I really wanted to run, but hadn't been able to because my left breast was still really sore from radiation. It felt bruised on the inside, and bouncing it about hurt. There was no rule against me walking during the triathlon, but my invigorating swims were motivating me to give running a try.

Chapter 15

Always the Victor,
Never the Victim

March 7. Saturday.

After an entire year of enduring the cure for breast cancer, I was back to my most prominent event of the year: the Los Angeles Marathon weekend. These races are extraordinary in their own right and already held a special place in my heart. But I felt uniquely excited to get back on my stages in LA because of what went down the year prior. If you remember, during the 2019 Los Angeles Marathon, all of our athletes went home with a gorgeous race medal and a long blonde Fitz hair. That finish line stage became the scene of one of the most challenging experiences of my life. However, being on that specific stage on that particular day was one of the greatest gifts I could have ever received. While my heart was breaking, I was surrounded by tens of thousands of people experiencing endless triumph and joy, which had filled my heart up. Being me at that moment was painful. Being there for them at that moment was a blessing. The ability to turn my focus away from my crisis and loudly celebrate others proved to be the one thing that kept me going all year long.

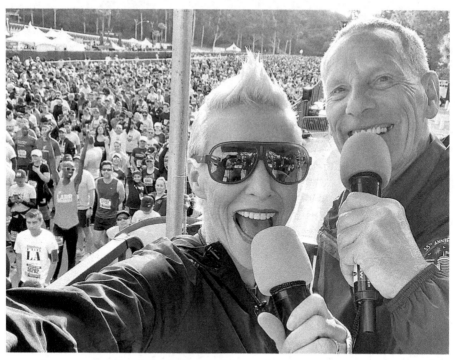

Sporting the shark fin at the start line of the LA Big 5k with Rudy.

Rudy and I climbed into our start line tower in front of Dodger Stadium around 6:30 a.m. for the LA Big 5K, which was set to begin at 8 a.m. The parking lot had already begun filling up with athletes who deserved some music and entertainment, which we were pleased to provide. Par for the course in LA, everyone showed up with a spunky attitude, and that included Team Noisy! The coronavirus, AKA COVID-19, had just started appearing in the United States, and since the threat of event cancellation was in the air, we were all fired up that these races were even taking place. I had created a newly-mixed race playlist and was totally gratified to see so many people dancing and bouncing to the beats as they lined up to start. Insider secret: spontaneous outdoor dancing at a non-dancing event is a sure sign that people are having fun.

Of the nearly 5,000 people who showed up for our 5K, at least a thousand or so were part of a team dedicated to raising awareness and funds for their favorite causes. Yes, there was quite a contingency of folks going the distance for cancer causes, but this race runs deep with variety. Some of the teams included:

- American Foundation for Suicide Prevention
- Connecting to Cure Crohn's and Colitis
- Big Brothers Big Sisters
- Gary Sinise Foundation
- Team Kitten Rescue!
- Team World Vision
- Angel City Pitbulls
- Special Olympics
- Train 4 Autism
- ARC

The list is far longer than I've shared, but you get the gist. I just wanted to demonstrate how genuinely generous, diverse, and productive the running community is. And again, when I say running community, I'm including people who exclusively walk. It's one of the reasons I work so hard to take such loving care of my athletes. They deserve it. My races are flooded with people doing positive things for their health, their communities, and worthy causes. That's why Rudy and I take them very seriously. We go above and beyond to recognize their causes, which are usually boldly written on their shirts. The other thing we did a lot of this weekend was recognize fans decked out in the jerseys of the late Kobe Bryant and his daughter, Gigi. This dynamic basketball duo had been killed in a helicopter crash only six weeks prior, and many were still grieving.

In 2019, even with the impending doom of baldness on the horizon, the joy our runners exuded as they crossed the LA Big 5K start line filled me with the good stuff. They did the same darn thing this year. Rudy yelled "GO," the whoopee parade ran by, and I felt deep satisfaction. Not only that I'd beaten breast cancer, but I felt so empowered that I never once allowed it to steal one second of my beloved profession from me. That stubborn mule that lives inside me kicked and bucked like a big noisy ass all damn year and proved to be my secret source of strength.

Was it hard? Yes! Was it scary and stressful? Absolutely! But in the end, I got to be the victor. I never once bowed down to cancer or played the role of victim. Not once. And because of that, I got to do things during treatment that no one imagined I could. All points awarded to … Fitz Koehler!

If you are wondering whether I actually did have this moment of satisfaction, the answer is "yes.". While all of our athletes were traipsing by waving, shouting, and celebrating, I was internally pumping my fist that I'd made it back in one piece. And that I was on my way to what should be a long, healthy life. Woohoo! I kept that to just a moment though, because partying with these people was the immediate item on my agenda.

Our finish line was just as engaging as the start, and I actually scored some goodies on my stage. An adorable duo of runners dressed up as Dodger stadium waiters ran the 5K carrying trays full of cotton candy, Cracker Jacks, and all other sorts of treats. As they ran through the finish, they tossed me a box of Red Vine licorice, which I love. Rudy and I also received doughnuts from a person dressed up as a doughnut. Who would think such silliness would take place at a running event? This type of thing actually happens a lot. And, speaking of silliness, I enjoyed endless amounts once I hustled over to announce the LA ½K Kids Races. Our athletes, ages eight and younger, brought boundless energy. Even though I told them that everyone who goes the distance would get a medal, they were revving their little engines eager to sprint the whole way. But first, and because it's tradition, we had ourselves a dance party. A few little boys showed up with similar hairstyles to mine and we took time to compare. My hair was styled into a fairly tall blonde spike, which I nicknamed my shark fin. The kids definitely dug it, and I stole from the popular Mommy Shark song to sing, "Noisy Shark, do doo do doo do doo!" Never thought I'd have a hairdo that was fun for kids, but I was making the best of it. When all of the cuties conquered their ½K, it was time to go rest up for the largest field of runners in the history of the Los Angeles Marathon.

March 8. Sunday.

I couldn't have wished for a better return to the Los Angeles Marathon. If you remember, in years past, I couldn't announce the start line with Rudy, because we needed to make sure someone was at the finish line early enough to congratulate our speedy hand cyclists. This year, one of our operations professionals, Toby Taylor, was assigned to fill in for me until I arrived at the finish. This enabled me to start my morning off with everyone else at Dodger Stadium. I can't tell you how delighted I was by this change. The start line is our opportunity to create a connection with our athletes. We're not just blah, blah, blah, reading a script. We're engaging, entertaining, and forming a legitimate relationship with each and every one of these people. Even amongst the masses, I feel like we get a bit of personal time with most of them. It makes our praise much more meaningful when we celebrate their accomplishments at the end. Getting to work the start meant way more than my directors, Kayla Newby-Fraser and Murphy Reinschreiber, could ever guess. Team Noisy arrived at the dark stadium at 4:30 a.m. and didn't yell "GO" for the first time until 6:30 a.m. But those two hours of action flew by. We had guidance to give, jokes to tell, and lots of personal friends to greet. It was a clear and cool morning around 50°F, and the high for that afternoon was 62°F. These were perfect conditions for a southern California marathon. The excitement intensified as busloads of athletes arrived, filling up the stadium parking lot. 27,000 runners registered for this marathon, and wrapped halfway around Dodger Stadium as they lined up to run from the "Stadium to the Sea."

Our start line itinerary was far stricter than usual because we were working closely with our media partner KTLA 5, who was broadcasting our event on live television. We're never willy-nilly about things, but the 20 minutes prior to our starts were micromanaged down to the very second. Everything on our schedule needed to mesh perfectly with the television broadcast. Some might have considered the situation stressful, but we felt like the added layer of detail just made things more exciting. But before the program became too tight, Rudy took the time to tell everyone about my battle with breast cancer and to introduce my new and improved shark fin hairdo. I appreciated the opportunity to give my most enormous audience of the year a brief synopsis. I figured it'd encourage them all to get their annual exams and squeeze their stuff. Gosh, I love how strongly the crowd responded. The crowd roared when I announced that my self-exam had saved my own life and that I had won my battle with cancer. And when I asked who was committed to squeezing their own stuff, the crowd roared even louder. Mission accomplished!

Once we hit that pre-race 20-minute mark, our tower started filling up with executives and dignitaries. Our honorary starters for the day (AKA air-horn-honkers) were Phil Shin, a liver cancer and transplant survivor, who was running the marathon and revered Dodger third baseman, Justin Turner. They were both thrilled to be in the tower and brought tons of radiant, positive energy. This event had so much grandiosity about it. The TV coverage of the start, finish, and heated competition on the course is pretty swanky. We had runners from all 50 states and 78 countries taking part and $100,000 in prize money to award. Helicopters hovered above us to cover it all and that's simply not something that happens at most races. We could feel the intensity, but that only fueled our chemistry and fun further. Rudy and I juggled bantering to keep our crowds entertained, managing our tightly scripted activities, and a TV producer giving directions and counting in our ears.

After introducing the dignitaries, the color guard, the choir of children singing God Bless America, and the national anthem, it was time for our athletes to start their proverbial engines. There would be five opportunities to yell, "Runners, seeeet" in LA. One for our hand cyclists, one for our racing chariots and push-rim chairs, one for the elite women, and then two for the masses. Rudy and I originally planned for me to launch the elite women, with him doing the rest. However, in his excitement, he forgot and launched the women's one too. Silly noisy man! That meant I got to launch the big wave, which I didn't mind at all. By the time we got to the 60-second warning for the grand majority of our runners pandemonium had struck Dodger stadium. Our call for jumping was heard and we once again presided over what looked like the largest mosh pit in history. With a couple of directors in my ear, I waited until

I heard, "10 seconds, 9, 8, 7, 6," and then I bellowed "Runners, Seeeet!" and Justin and Phil slammed on their air horns at precisely 6:55 a.m. Glorious organized chaos ensued.

With a juiced-up version of Randy Newman's song, "I Love L.A." blaring from the speakers, there wasn't a more invigorating place in the entire world to be. It's thrilling to see tens of thousands of the most lively and athletic people from around the world leap for joy in front of you. The fact that a grand percentage of them are looking up at us, calling our names, waving, shouting, and blowing kisses, just felt surreal.

And while I was truly having the time of my life, at 7 a.m. sharp, I received a tap on my shoulder. Our VP, Murphy, was summoning me to go. Like Cinderella when the clock struck midnight, I was about to turn into a pumpkin if I didn't leave. That was our deal. I could announce the start, only if I agreed to leave and go straight to the finish line with him at 7 a.m. Although I was sad to be leaving the party before it was over, that sorrow was completely washed over by the extreme gratification I felt for the great majority of the morning. The only thing left to do was watch, wave, and cheer for the next 20,000 runners as they cruised by, which is pretty dang fun.

I'd like to point out that I avoid referring to my profession as work whenever possible. Sure, I make money announcing races and teaching fitness, but I just can't bring myself to minimize something I love so much and that fulfills my passion so profoundly. Calling it work would feel disparaging, so I've spent the past three decades finding other words for it. Profession. Career. Calling. Passion. They all suffice in a way that work never would. I wish everyone earned a living doing something they loved so much. Before I descended from our tower, Rudy and I shared a big happy hug for our job-well done. He was just as excited as I was that we were able to be together at the start. I hustled to Murphy's fancy ride, and we headed to Santa Monica for more noisy fun at the finish line.

The timing was perfect, and I arrived at the finish line before any of our hand cyclists. In fact, our first wheeled athletes didn't show up for another 20 minutes. Toby was ready and waiting at the microphone though, so I shared my appreciation for his efforts with a hug. He's a team player, and I feel fortunate to work with him and call him a friend. Our new audio company brought big sound and quality customer service, which totally made up for the debacle the year prior. Things were going my way. To be honest, everything went my way that day. And Team Noisy's way. And the Los Angeles Marathon's way. The entire day was phenomenal from start to finish. The weather was picture-perfect, our team was firing on all cylinders, 6,000-plus generous volunteers had swarmed our course to provide support, and our athletes brought gargantuan enthusiasm to our finish line. Rudy and I spent the entire day dancing, laughing, and sending love from above.

Nothing is more rewarding to us than when our runners allow themselves to celebrate their accomplishments and truly enjoy the culmination of their efforts. The finish line of a marathon doesn't just signify the most recent 26.2 miles conquered. It signifies the months or years of training and preparation that were required to even get to the start line. It's the reward for waking up absurdly early to get in some training miles before work, skipping happy hour in pursuit of proper nutrition, and spending hard-earned money on travel, hotel, and race registrations. Finish lines are often life-changing, and this one in particular demands a raucous response. When you come through the finish line of the Los Angeles Freaking Marathon, you have a moral obligation to get a little crazy and allow yourself a bold and unconstrained celebration.

One of the things I'm most grateful for is my ability to emotionally let go and get past the bad stuff. Sure, my experience at the 2019 Los Angeles Marathon was trying. Of course, I didn't like losing much of my hair there. But clenching on to that memory and harping on it long-term wasn't going to benefit me in any way, shape, or, form. At no point did I stand there on my stage, conjuring up sad visions of hair everywhere. What good would that have done? Will I ever forget? Probably not. But will I let these bad experiences cloud my future good ones? Not a chance.

Folks, the point of spending this year fighting for my life was so I could live. Truly live. While I was brutalized by the process at times, I did not allow cancer to interfere with my special family engagements or the pursuit of the career of my dreams. I will go forward, choosing not to carry the lousy memories on my back or in my heart. I will not live like cancer has created a long-term sentence for me. I WAS weak. I WAS sick. When my treatment concludes, my plan is to get back to being full-force Fitz Koehler as quickly as possible. Then I will then double down and become twice as strong as the girl I lost when I found my lump.

Having breast cancer wasn't my choice. Beating the hell out of it was. I've chosen not to allow that nasty disease to occupy any more space on my body or in my mind. No ribbons. No tattoos. I have firmly decided that I will only address this thing on my terms, in a way that makes me better, and that benefits those around me. I will spend the rest of my life looking over my shoulder and hoping it won't be back. But I will not spend the rest of my life, allowing my past to drag me down.

When 3 p.m. rolled around, and our sound system was unplugged, Rudy and I climbed down from our tower feeling mighty satisfied. The entire weekend had been sensational, and we felt particularly rewarded by the magnitude of merriment we were able to invoke along the way. We left our seaside stage and walked over to California Pizza Kitchen for food and relaxation. Unlike in 2019, this year there were no tears. Instead, our booth was filled with laughter and fond memories of good times and great people.

March 10. Tuesday.

My flight home landed around 10 p.m. the previous night, so I wasn't exactly thrilled when my 7 a.m. alarm went off. However, I had a 7:45 a.m. appointment for a mammogram and ultrasound, and I was pretty eager to get both. My December PET scan was clear, but it had been four months, and I wanted to know if there was or wasn't anything nefarious going on inside my chest. I'm proud to reveal that Dr. Yancey found absolutely nothing to write home about. My boobs were just regular boobs, and even though I wasn't stressed when I walked into her office, I sure did feel incredible relief when I walked out.

I left that appointment and made a beeline to swim laps at the gym. I then returned home so Rob could drive me to FCS for Godzilla. Round #18. Life as a human yo-yo was still very weird. Going from the high point of race announcing to the low point of having drugs pumped into me through my port was very strange indeed. However, the highs kept me motivated, and thankfully, the lows I was experiencing weren't so low anymore. My appointments were kind of upbeat at this point, because nurse John was super silly and sarcastic, and my side effects were no longer too harsh. All I was really left with was some fatigue and a few food aversions.

March 20. Friday.

I was supposed to start my day off by flying to Tempe, Arizona, to announce the DC Wonder Woman Run Series. Goodness, I was so excited to get back into my tutu and tiara. Unfortunately, the world was making different plans. As the coronavirus (COVID-19) spread from country to country, including the United States, all events where large groups of people gathered were being canceled. Within just a few days, I was notified by a handful of race directors that 17 of my events had been canceled. Several others were postponed. SEVENTEEN EVENTS! More cancelations would come. Ugh! Folks, for the very last time, I'm going to re-reference those best-laid plans. I was over the moon about my spring and summer races. As I said at the start, I do believe I have the absolute best race announcing schedule in this business. Chemo's effects on me the year prior were savage, and I gave every ounce of my being toward fighting through it. I didn't miss one single event. And now that I was starting to feel better ... Poof! It all disappeared.

And this, my friends, is why perspective is my best friend. Sure, if I whined or moaned, some might find it justifiable. But then again, what good would it do? None. Where would it get me? Nowhere. And how downright annoying would it be to everyone around me? Very. So I decided to just be grateful to be alive. The reality that my year could have gone very differently was and still is front and center in my mind. I am fortunate to be mostly healthy, and I was going to focus on making the best of this forced downtime. I'd schmooze with my cool family, exercise, and put some effort into finishing this book. My rule of thumb is to control what I can and get past the things I cannot. This societal shutdown fell under the second category.

March 31. Tuesday.

Thanks to that virus everyone loves to hate, I went in for chemo #19 all by my lonesome. FCS wouldn't allow anyone who wasn't essential to patient care to enter the infusion room. So, Rob drove me to my appointment and walked me through the big lobby, but then we parted ways. If you're wondering why he was still driving me, it's because the Benadryl and anti-nausea meds I was given through my IV made me tired and loopy. I was functional, but not safe to drive.

Without Rob's hand to squeeze during the big needle stick in my chest, I told my nurse John that he had to be extra nice to me. He's always really nice, but I love giving him a hard time. Oh! And here's a funny little tidbit. A few weeks prior, I had posted a photo of John, my beautiful friend Linda Bennett, and myself in the infusion room. Linda is in the process of torching ovarian cancer, and we enjoyed being with each other during chemo. Back to the photo, though. The response to John was pretty fantastic. Gobs of gals were commenting that they wished they had some sort of minor ailment that would allow them to go get some attention from John. He's a total hunk, so it was all well-deserved. More importantly, the man had been giving me very fancy Sugar Skull bandages to cover my port when I was done with chemo. This made me feel like I did when my pediatrician gave me cool stickers or allowed me to pick a prize out of the treasure chest. Sugar Skull bandages became very exciting, indeed.

Fitzness Log

On March 1st, I threw on my snuggest most-supportive sports bra, stepped onto a treadmill, cranked it up to five miles per hour, and ran exactly one-quarter of a mile. The distance was intentionally tiny, as I wanted this experience to yield only good feelings. I'm smart enough to start small, very small, and progress slowly without letting ego interfere. That would be the ticket to my long term success.

Every few days, I would return to the treadmill and add on a quarter-mile. It made my boob slightly sore, but not in a way that would deter me anymore. One of the things I love most about running is that it makes me feel like I'm five years old. It can definitely become challenging, but for the most part, I find it freeing. After spending a year fighting for my life, it felt good to feel youthful and vibrant again. I was now swimming, walking, running, strength training, and stretching. On the comeback for sure!

Chapter 16

Give Me a "C" (The Other C)

April 20. Monday.

Before I sat down for chemo round #20, I went in for my scheduled appointment with Dr. Gordan. Rob still wasn't allowed to join me because of the annoying COVID-19 restrictions. Instead, he joined us via speakerphone. I hadn't seen Dr. Gordan since January, so I was looking forward to it. He walked into my room, all bundled up in his white coat, gloves, and mask. I could still see him smiling with his eyes and he greeted me warmly referencing air hugs. After a few niceties about how much he liked my hair, we got to the good stuff.

Dr. Gordan was satisfied with my results and more than confident I was unlikely to face a recurrence. There are various types of breast cancer, and I was in one of the categories with the most hopeful long-term expectations. He also took the time to praise the healthy behaviors that helped me through this experience. He said that while he knew I suffered tremendously, if I hadn't been so healthy, things would have been a lot worse. I could have been hospitalized more often or dealt with complications like pneumonia.

Most importantly, he used the "C" word. Not the scary one he started with, cancer. He used the amazing one declaring he believed I was CURED! I wanted to leap into his arms and give him a mammoth squeeze, but pouncing on my wizard of a doctor would simply have to be postponed. Damn you, COVID-19. Rob and I thanked him profusely for literally saving my life, and then Dr. Gordan posed for a few super smiley selfies with me.

It's funny. At the beginning it was very hard to believe that I actually had cancer. Wrapping my head around that concept was very difficult. And now, it's been somewhat difficult to believe that I no longer have cancer. Dr. Sarantos

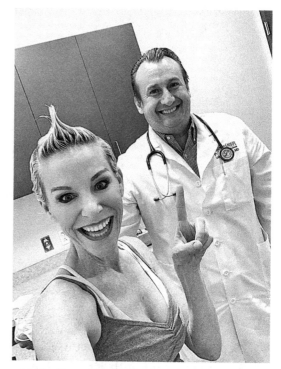

My brilliant oncologist, Dr. Lucio Gordan.

removed any known cancer from my body during surgery on July 30th. Technically that's when I went into complete remission. Many scans have been clean and I've shown what they call "No Evidence of Disease" since. However, I didn't shout it from the rooftops. I did tell my family and a few close friends, of course. But I felt like I needed to be patient and see several levels of proof that my cancer was really gone before sharing with the world. It'd been almost nine months since surgery, and there were zero signs of trouble. I finally felt confident and comfortable that I had beaten the beast!

Back for chemo #20 I went. Feeling happy, healthy, and energetic, I bounced through the infusion room toward my nurse John, with a huge shit-eating grin on my face. I wondered if the other patients thought I was annoying or wonderful, but I couldn't have wiped the elation off of my face if I tried. It stunk that Rob couldn't be there with me, but John poured on the silliness and his fellow nurse Tammy kept things light. I left chemo with another fancy Sugar Skull bandage over my port and was grateful I only had one left. I could finally see the light at the end of the tunnel.

Fitzness Log

While the world had shut down, including the Gainesville Health and Fitness Center, I was still hell-bent on becoming fitter. I was sad that I no longer had access to either the lap pool or my neighborhood pool, but where there's a will, there's a way. Instead of giving up, I pivoted. During quarantine, Rob bought me a $98.00 mountain bike at Walmart and I began riding. I could only go a few miles at a time because the dang hills in my neighborhood set my legs on fire. I struggled to get over the fairly small hills and completely bonked trying to climb killer hill. In fact, I failed. Once I'd ride past the third house on my street, I'd have to dismount and walk my bike home. Did I feel like a failure? No way. I felt like a woman on a mission. I loved that my bike rides nearly made me hyperventilate. It was a sign that I was challenging my body and making it fitter all the time.

The other thing I returned to was climbing the bleachers at The Swamp, the UF football stadium. Imagine a massive football stadium built to hold 100,000 fans completely empty, with the exception of you and a handful of other people trying to get in a killer workout. Some people run up and down the actual steps in a serpentine pattern around the whole thing. I choose to walk up and down the steep bleacher seats to get a much more focused glute and quad workout. This workout is a bear, but that's what I wanted. With each step I took toward row 90, I was building my bodacious booty back up. And I was also pumping up my heart and lungs. "No more chemo butt for me," I thought. During my first visit, I climbed three flights and left to walk around the campus. During my second visit, I climbed six flights. Continuously going back to do equal or more than I'd done before would be the secret to my success. By the end of April, I was doing 12 flights per workout. I was scheduled for a Spartan obstacle course 5K race in June. And this time I wasn't announcing it. I was running it.

On the nutrition side of things, I was able to start eating big salads and veggies like cauliflower, broccoli, peppers, squash, and carrots without consequences. My stomach wasn't completely normal, but it was getting there. Being able to enjoy a greater variety of fresh healthy foods was really exciting.

Chapter 17

Celebrating My Finish Line

May 11. Monday.

For the first time ever, I woke up excited about chemo. Well, not really about chemo itself, but I was thrilled that the poisoning was finally coming to the end. The 15 months since my diagnosis had been absolutely daunting, and moving past both cancer and life as a cancer patient was something I was eager to do. However, it was all still surreal. All of it. Looking back, I still can't believe that I had cancer, chemo, surgery, and radiation! The thought of sitting down for my final chemo was as confusing as sitting down for my first. It was almost impossible to wrap my head around. But, I was definitely stoked about getting it over with. Rob still wasn't allowed into the infusion room, so our big plan was for him to drop me off and then pick me up with the kids. Ginger and I were going to record another celebratory dance using the TikTok app. That was it.

I worked hard to contain my emotions as I checked in. Even though I was about to take a wonderful step forward, there continued to be stress in my situation. Not the terrifying stress that I had at the start, but more like the kind that comes with ... relief? I say that with a question mark because I can't explain my feelings all the way. I can just tell you that I had to fight to avoid blubbering like a baby in that lobby. Alan checked me in and I bid Rob adieu as I headed back alone. It was a shame. Rob had been there for all of the awful appointments. It would have been wonderful if he could have joined me for this good one. As my nurse John poked the big needle through my chest for the last time, I cursed aloud as I had done during all of the previous pokes. I did take pleasure in the fact that (hopefully) nobody would ever do that to me again. I was also pleased to refuse Benadryl. If I had an allergic reaction on my final day, I didn't care. I wouldn't need Godzilla anymore anyway. Thanks to that decision, I didn't walk out of the building like a sleepy zombie. The chemo itself would force me into bed all week, but I didn't have the same instant fatigue I normally experienced.

Even though I was bubbling over with joy, the busy infusion room was unusually quiet, so I made a concerted effort not to be annoying to the other cancer patients around me. I remembered all too well what it was like to feel like death warmed over. Instead, I sat fairly quietly and counted the minutes until my high-tech IV contraption would beep to signal that I was done. I also imagined how fabulous it would be if my hair instantly grew out to its original length upon completion of chemo. You know. I'd hear a big "BOOP!" sound and spontaneously have long golden locks again. And I would also regain my still-absent nostril hair. It would have been a pretty cool phenomenon if that happened, but no such luck.

Thirty minutes after my Godzilla drip started, it stopped. And my IV machine beeped, signalling the completion of my last bag of chemo. In the past, that incessant beeping sound was often pretty annoying. This time, it sounded beautiful. In fact, I heard the IV machine proclaim, "Here ye! Here ye! You are done with this nightmare! Please go forth, live long, and live happily!" Nurse John zipped on over to my chair, un-hooked the tubes, and removed the needle from my chest. Another fancy Sugar Skull bandage was applied and it was finally time to party. Now, partying in the infusion room is pretty tame. I had seen it happen many times throughout my treatment though, and I was eagerly awaiting my turn. Remember, I rang the bell when I completed radiation. At the completion of chemo at FCS, patients get a little disco party. And I was ready for mine. All it really entailed was John turning on the stereo to play Kool and the Gang's song "Celebration" as a little disco ball sprayed speckled lights around the ceiling tiles. Technically there wasn't anyone to celebrate with, per se, but it was MY lame little disco party. And I was totally into it. I sprang from my chair, went over to John's workstation to be closer to the music and lights, and I danced. All alone. Like a very happy, little cancer-free nerd. John and the other nurses let out a few "woohoos" and boogied a bit while they cared for the other patients. For the most part, it was just me and I was totally okay with that. My cancer. My care. My cure. My party. But I wasn't alone for long.

When the song end-ed, John gathered a "Fi-nal Chemo" sign that he wrote May 11th on with a dry erase marker and es-corted me out to meet my family in the lobby. I was greeted with happy hugs and love from Rob, Gin-ger, and Parker. They gave me pretty balloons Kim Cinque had dropped off and we took a bunch of photos with John before he returned to work. I will always be grateful for the loving care I received from John and my first chemo nurse, Lilly. They genuinely made my life better. Before we left the lobby, Ginger and I set up my phone to perform our chemo completion dance

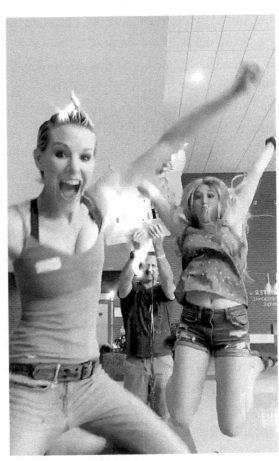

Screenshot from my celebratory dance with Ginger.

to The Weeknd's song "Blinding Lights". It was only a 16 second routine, but it was crazy fun, and a wonderful way to put a bow on my treatment. It included a bit of running, jumping, big arm circles, and a giant leap at the end. Like our radiation celebration dance video, this was viewed by tens of thousands of people.

I had texted Rob about going to lunch after chemo and thought we had agreed to do so. But as we drove out of the medical complex, he turned toward home instead of the restaurant. I tried to correct him, but he told me that Parker wasn't feeling well and that we should go out to dinner instead. I was fairly surprised and disappointed, but thought, "Oh well. Fine!" It was strange that they weren't doing this simple thing for me, but as all moms will attest, our needs are often put on the backburner. I can't tell you how surprised I was when we pulled into my neighborhood and saw dozens and dozens of neighbors lining the streets, holding beautiful hand-made signs, and cheering. For me. Seriously. My heart leaped out of my chest and my eyes filled up with tears. It was absolutely heartwarming. I rolled down my window and shouted "thank you" and "I love you" to everyone we passed. I wanted to stop the car, get out, and hug them all. But the awkwardness due to social distancing rules prevented me from doing so. That is until I saw my long-time friend and neighbor, Leah Galione, whom I knew had organized the entire thing. I don't know if Rob told me or if I just guessed. But I broke the rules for her and gave her a ginormous hug. We cried a bit together too. I loved every second of that drive down the long road. When we hit the end, I wanted to go back to see everyone, but Rob drove me home instead. Waiting for me were more friends and neighbors, more signs, and more cheering. And then, almost all of the neighbors from the main street started walking up killer hill to our home. That's when it all became too much. The tears came out and I spent a few moments buckled over in the middle of the road. Alas, it was finally over. And I felt it. The weight of breast cancer had finally been lifted off of my chest (literally), and we had a legitimate reason to celebrate. As my neighbors flooded my front yard with their signs, balloons, and adorable pinwheels, I felt a deep sense of appreciation. Their artwork was cheerful, personal, and funny. And the

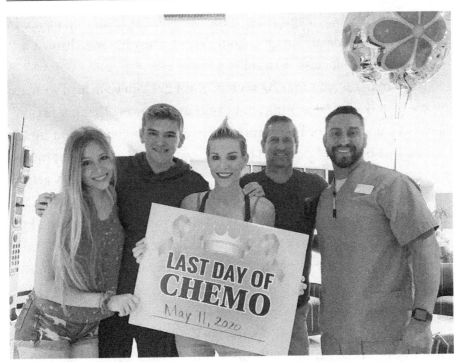

With my family and nurse, John. 21 rounds of chemo and done!

colorful spinning pinwheels brought real life to my home. I had no interest in telling them that they shouldn't have. Getting to live was a proper reason to celebrate and I loved every minute of it. Once they all returned to their homes, the Koehlers headed to a Mexican restaurant for lunch. My meal was delicious and I'm happy to say that there was absolutely no black dirt on my food.

I have to be honest. On many days, it felt like my treatment would never end. That the sickness, fatigue, pain, soreness, baldness, and stress would never go away. Of course, it eventually would, but my time in purgatory did not fly by as many had suggested. Standing here on the other side of breast cancer, I'm elated to feel like me again. I'm writing this passage one week after completing my treatment. I'm 80% of who I was and I am in hot pursuit of attaining full-force Fitz Koehler status again. I loved her and can't wait to be her! Along the way, many have declared that this was all happening for a reason. I vehemently disagree. I don't think I was chosen for some sick and demented game of "Fight for your

Life!" I don't think a magic man in the sky pointed at me and planted a seed of doom. Instead, I'm quite confident that my life was thrown into a whirlwind by one nasty bastard of a rogue cell.

Now, many of you may be saying "But Fitz! You've helped so many people by talking and writing about your experiences. That *is* a reason!" Nope. It's not. Do not be confused. There was no good reason for my cancer. Just because I pounced on some opportunities does not mean I was predestined for it. I reject that suggestion on all levels. My actions are a result of who I am despite cancer, not because of it. In fact, I'm frequently asked if fighting cancer has led me to any revelations, the kind of life-altering epiphanies that would make me change directions. I'm proud to say that the opposite is true. This experience has completely solidified my foundation. More than ever, I'm committed to my chosen profession and the people I care about. There was a reason I wasn't willing to press pause on race announcing, The Morning Mile, my Fitzness business, or special times with my family. It was already that good. I used to believe I was unstoppable, and I'm happy to report that I am back to feeling the same way. Although, I am clearly capable of being slowed down dramatically.

As with all dark clouds, there were silver linings. The amount of kindness generated toward myself and my family this year has been unfathomable. On many occasions, it felt as though everyone in the world had our back. Old friends, new friends, and many people who I didn't even know, came out of the woodwork to pitch in or send kind words. I was gifted with warm blankets, cozy socks, inspiring bracelets, moisturizers, hats, buffs, gift baskets, flowers, chocolate-covered fruit, custom-made clothing, books, house cleaning services, gift cards, healthy meals, and more. A constant stream of thoughtful cards and letters landed in my mailbox every week. Strangers went out of their way to take care of the bald girl with simple acts of chivalry, kind words, bonus cookies, and of course, that lucky rock. If everyone experienced as much kindness and support in their entire life as I was granted during this 15-month ordeal, the world would be a much better place.

Now more than ever, I am excited about my own health and motivated to become incredibly fit again. I'm also even more passionate about YOUR health. Folks, I appreciate you taking the time to read my story. I hope you enjoyed going on this rollercoaster ride with me. But I would be remiss if I didn't finish up by turning the tables on you. As you can see, health, mobility, and longevity aren't guarantees. They're rewards. If you don't put in a certain amount of effort toward those things, you can't expect to have them. Yes, I was healthy and yes, I got cancer. It can happen to anyone. However, I got cancer and I kicked its royal ass while ricocheting around the country and having more fun than most healthy people experience in a decade. I never missed a professional event, nor did I miss one single opportunity to support my kids as they played sports, performed on stages, or experienced other special moments. If I weren't so incredibly healthy going into this nightmare, I might not be able to make those claims. In fact, I'm pretty sure I would have been homebound. Without living in fear, I deem it wise to constantly prepare your body for battle and recovery. A strong, flexible body with quality heart and lung capacity will endure any sort of crisis far more easily than an unfit one. And, when faced with trauma, it will be far more capable of rebounding at a much faster pace.

Moving forward, I plan to savor every healthy day I'm granted and pursue active adventure like never before. I will continue to love my people all the way and make as much happy noise as humanly possible.

Plug your ears, because I. AM. BACK!

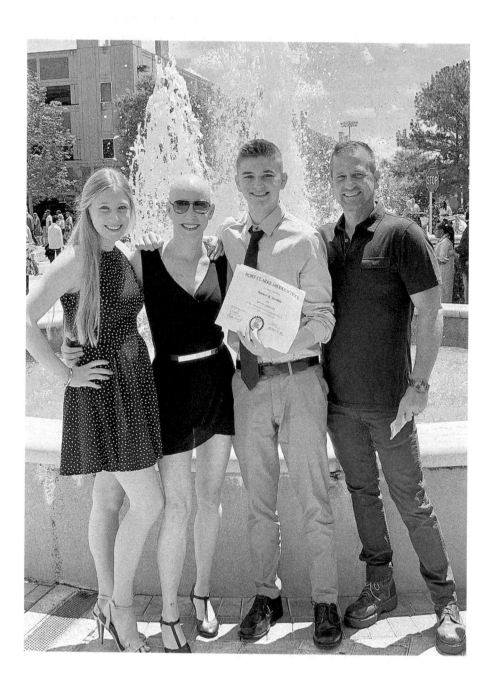

Acknowledgements

Rob. Thank you for taking extraordinary care of me throughout this nightmare. You helped me stand, walk, eat, drink, sleep, travel, endure pokes and hospitals, and I couldn't have survived any of it without you.

Ginger Bean. Thank you for holding my hand on walks, coaxing me into doing silly TikTok dances, frequently hugging me, occasionally crying with me, and making me laugh often. You are brave, bold, stunningly beautiful, and the most delightful human on earth. You are the sunshine.

Parker Beans. From the second you told me that I'd be cute bald, I breathed a sigh of relief. Thank you for your healing hugs, mitten-style hand-holding, and long thoughtful talks. I'm amazed that one person could be so athletic, artistic, insightful, cuddly, and funny all at the same time. My Pooh!

Piper. My loyal best friend. You never left my side. Thank you for protecting me and caring for me with your cuddles and kisses.

Handy. You stole my heart the second you laid your sweet little head in my hand. You brought me so much joy and comfort and I will always cherish the time when you were mine.

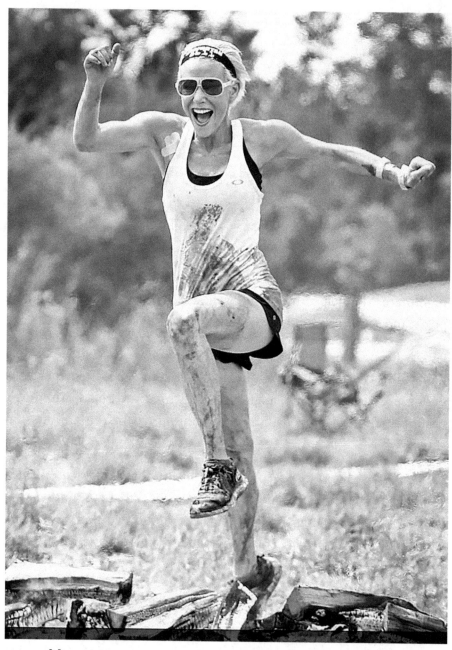

My port came out June 3rd. I ran the Spartan 5k on June 13th.
Photo by Spartan.

Mom. Sorry to put you through this. Thank you for making me, raising me right, and visiting so much.

John. You're the best big brother in the world and, while I loathed being bald, I really enjoyed being bald with you. Let's go adventuring together soon.

Rudy Novotny. You were often my home away from home and having you by my side was exactly what I needed. Thanks for leading me into race announcing and for your endless support along the way. You're the best noisy friend and partner I could ask for.

Cheryl Tyrone. Thank you for your friendship, for your guidance, for the referrals to outstanding physicians, for organizing the Meal Train, and for sharing your farm family. Also, thanks for allowing John to continue obnoxiously posting on social media. He makes me laugh daily.

Helen Legall. You went out of your way to support me while still fighting your own breast cancer battle, and I never took that for granted. After your distinguished career as a police officer, you deserve nothing but peace, health, and happiness.

Jennifer Senn. Thank you for homemade soup, custom-made fuzzy hats, cookies that lasted a year, rides for my kids, visits to chemo, walks, talks, and more. Your giving never stops and you genuinely made my life easier on a regular basis. And thank you for your edits!

Arup Senn. Your concoctions are magical and I'm proud to be "fueled by Fluffy!"

Nicole Zimmerman Bodlack. We've been friends since elementary school, and we'll be friends forevermore. Thank you for loving me, bringing me sweet gifts, sitting with me at chemo, driving my groggy tush around, and for the easy girl-time.

Kim Cinque, the Patron Saint of Gainesville. Your generosity is endless, and our entire community benefits because of it. Thank you for the rides,

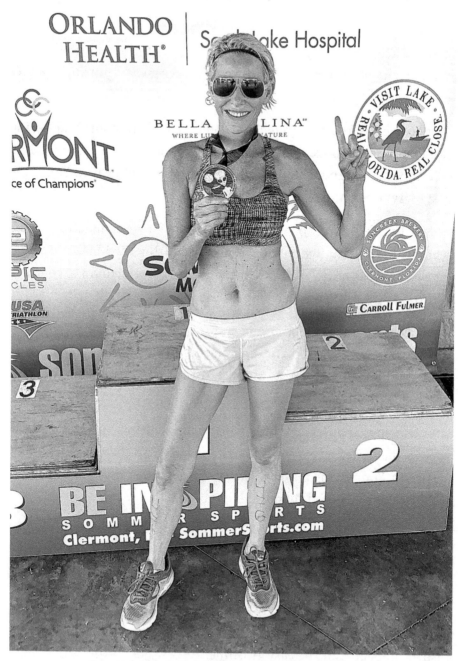

I completed a mini sprint triathlon on June 27th.
Finished dead last and proud!

chemo visits, and lunch dates. Can't wait to return to your Gator tailgates and share a couple of beers!

Anne Lowry, thank you for bringing Deux by during my chemo infusions for cuddles and kisses. His "service" to me was real, and allowing him to break protocol made me feel very special!

Heather and Mark Scheel. Thank you for driving Parker so often and for including him in your fun family.

Jo and Bill McFarland, thank you for driving Ginger so often and for the hand-made fuzzy hats!

My race directors. Greg Weber, Eva Solomon, Gary Kutscher, Doug Thurston, Mark Knutson, Beth Salinger, Rich Clark, Christine Adams, Robert Wells, Jonathan Sykes, Ryan Jordan, Keith Jordan, Murphy Reinschreiber, Tracey Russell, Bob Nichols, Meg Nichols, Kelsey Beall, Jodi Book, Lisa Scolman, Leo Dignam, Greg Mislick, and Buddy Sharp. Your faith that I could and would continue to perform at my best throughout my treatment meant everything. The threat of losing even one of my beloved events weighed heavily on me and would have proved to be a crushing loss during an already difficult time. You stuck with me and provided me with the opportunity to forget I was sick for a while and bask in the joy of our races and runners. I adore serving you, your events, and our athletes. I consider you all dear friends and am so very lucky to have each of you in my life.

Rob Middaugh. My weekly physical therapy appointments with you are what kept me upright and physically functional … and laughing. You're a master of your craft and I wish I could take you everywhere I go. Mostly, I need to thank your evil thumbs. My armpits hate them, but the rest of me thinks they're great.

Deeta Adkins, my massage therapist, acupuncturist, and friend. We've been through so much over the past 16 years and you've always had a solution for the ridiculous things I've done to make my body cranky. You're a genius with your hands and talking to you for hours each month

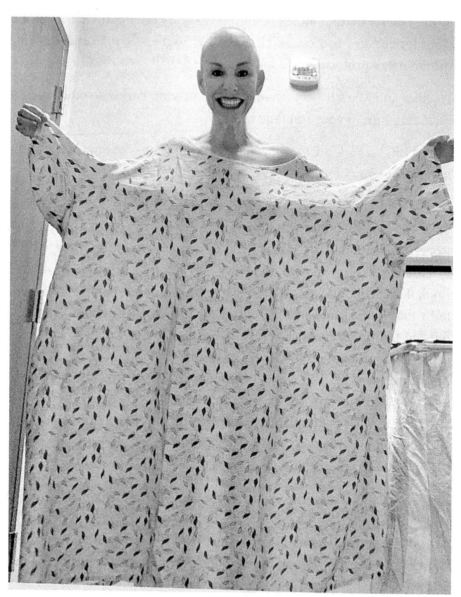

The big yellow gowns were fun!

is the cherry on top. Even though I curse at you and threaten to kill you regularly, I sincerely love you.

Ginger and Parker's Teachers! Thank you for your compassion and extra support. Your understanding that kids suffer when a highly involved mother becomes debilitated, was a lifesaver.

My doctors! Hand-picking people to save your life is a pretty big deal. And when it came to cancer care, there is no way I was going to settle for less than the best. I couldn't be more pleased with the team of physicians I chose to save me.

Dr. Lucio Gordan. You led me through the most difficult part of my treatment and having you at the helm gave me faith that the struggle was worth it. Thank you for saving my life with calm yet confident care.

Dr. Cherryle Hayes. You are the razor blade. Everything about you is wicked sharp, and I love that you wrap that big brain of yours in a huge smile, a stylish wardrobe, and endless sassiness. Thank you for saving my life with your zaps.

Dr. Peter Sarantos. You held my hands and looked into my eyes while promising I would be okay. And I believed you. Thank you for saving my life with your surgical skills.

Lilly Stoll. You made chemo far less terrifying and far more comfortable. You cared for me, comforted me, and protected me. And I love you for it. Thank you for the celebratory dance too!

John Colon. You made me laugh while rudely poking needles into my chest! You were a sweetie pie when I was super sick and made chemo kind of fun when I was on the mend. Your observation skills, well, they need work!

Kristi Hill. Thank you for being my incessant source of laughter. You're the funnest BFF I could ever ask for and I know you have my back. Fun-pig, this Noisy Mannequin will love you forever.

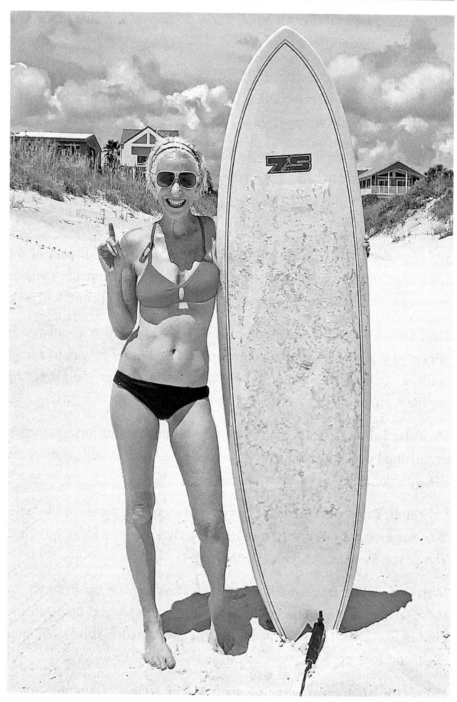

Picked up surfing in July. Lots of living to do!

My Big Sur Family. Doug, Chris, Sally, Hillary, Christy, Thompson, Joe, Hugo, Karen, Cath, Tom, Tino, Claudia, Dave, Heidi, Shirley, Sharon, Kevin, Julie, Hank, Bill, Ben the supermodel, Alice, Blake, Greg, Buddy, Bob, Megan, Toula, John, Wayne, Becky, Ute and Kecia …. Twice a year is never enough.

The ladies of LAE. Kelley, Taylor, Judy, and Sammie. You helped me feel like the best version of myself. I'm so grateful for your service and friendship.

Creigh Kelley and Jay Sutherland. I appreciate your extra efforts to support me and this book.

Toby Taylor and Mike Haughey. Thank you for the chivalry and care at our races. Sunscreen, water, chocolate milk, snacks, and hugs. You two make me feel like I've got big brothers on race day. And I love it.

My pool squad. Marty, Glen, Dan, Nestle, Ruth, Ann and Willie. The greatest soggy fitness friends in Gainesville.

Joe Cirulli. Thank you for building state of the art fitness facilities in our small town. The Gainesville Health and Fitness Center provided me with everything I needed to return to being me. You're a genius, a gentleman, and a dear friend. Thank you for your endless support and the case of chocolate milk!

All law enforcement officers, first responders, military personnel, and veterans. You had nothing to do with my cancer battle, but I will never miss an opportunity to thank you for protecting freedom and for your service to this extraordinary country. Your sacrifice is selfless, and I appreciate each and every one of you.

Beta Readers! Thanks for making this book better.

My Hotties. I love your commitment to health, your grit, your sweaty selfies, and your support of each other. Thank you for trusting me to guide you and for allowing me to be a part of your success. I'm endlessly proud of you. Michael Jones, thank you for leading the charge when I couldn't. #noexcuses

My runners. To the millions I've had the honor of serving at races, thank you! Thank you for showing up in pursuit of athletic adventure while caring for your health, your communities, and great causes. I learned at a young age that I should always associate up, and I can always do that when I'm with you. I adore waking up far too early to gather with you and send you on your way. Know that once I yell "GO", and you leave the start area, I always miss you and anxiously await your return at the finish line. You've inspired me with your grittiness, passion, creativity, friendships, costumes, celebrations, tears, kindness, compassion, and power. Without our time together during my treatments, I would have been lost. I hope we can agree that you'll keep showing up to race, and I'll keep showing up to make sure you're properly entertained and adored.

My fellow race professionals. You are the most rugged, positive, ambitious, inventive, and caring group of professionals on Earth. Your ability to avert crisis at 2 a.m. on a Sunday with little more than a few traffic cones and zip ties is extraordinary. It's a privilege to work at your side and I love getting to be a part of the magic you create.

Mike and Andy Reilly. Thank you both for the generous guidance on the self-publishing process. Like father, like son. I'm grateful to have you both as colleagues and friends. Mike, I hope to share a stage with you someday.

Neighbors. We're so lucky to live in a place with so many kind and thoughtful people. Your support was constant and the welcome home parade after my last round of chemo made me feel incredibly loved and special. Thank you!

Marilyn. You are beautiful, sexy, funny, and the most fabulous girl on Instagram. Our cancer sucked, but at least we got each other out of it. I love you and hope to come hug you in Israel someday.

Lily Ascher. Thank you for the thoughtful handmade gifts and cards, and for baking me so many treats.

My world of friends. Thank you for the care, concern, kind messages, meals, thoughtful gifts, prayers, laughs, and — above all — love.

UP NEXT:

YOUR HEALTHY CANCER COMEBACK

. . .

About the Author

Fitz Koehler, M.S.E.S.S. is one of the most prominent and compelling fitness experts and race announcers in America. As the voice of the Los Angeles Marathon, Philadelphia Marathon, Big Sur Marathon, DC Wonder Woman Run Series, and more, she brings big structure, energy, and joy to sport. She's also passionate about guiding others to live better and longer through her company, Fitzness®. Fitz has appeared on national media outlets and has worked as a speaker and spokesperson for corporations like Disney® and Office Depot®. She has also inspired millions of kids to get active through her successful school running/walking program, The Morning Mile®. Fitz enjoys water sports, strength training, animals, hugs, sarcasm, and travel. She lives in Gainesville, Florida with her husband and two kids.

FITZNESS.COM®

Visit Fitzness.com for guidance on living better and longer.
Pro tip: Start by reading The Exact Formula for Weight Loss!

Listen to Fitz's podcast The Fitzness Show, available on iTunes,
Audible, Spotify, and more.

Subscribe to the Fitzness channel on YouTube for instructional
workout videos and other fun fitness content.

Order the FLIP FLOP ABS core training DVD at Fitzness.com

Book Fitz to speak at your next event or announce your next race.

Follow Fitz on Facebook and Instagram @Fitzness

fitzness.com

facebook

instagram

CPSIA information can be obtained
at www.ICGtesting.com
Printed in the USA
LVHW080228011020
667596LV00010B/1907